LIFE
after
PSYCHOTHERAPY

LIFE after PSYCHOTHERAPY

Todd Davison, M.D.

JASON ARONSON INC.
Northvale, New Jersey
London

This book was set in 11 pt. New Century Schoolbook by Alpha Graphics of Pittsfield, New Hampshire, and printed and bound by Book-mart Press, Inc. of North Bergen, New Jersey.

Copyright © 1997 by Todd Davison, M.D.

10 9 8 7 6 5 4 3 2 1

All rights reserved. No part of this book may be used or reproduced in any manner whatsoever without written permission from Jason Aronson Inc. except in the case of brief quotations in reviews for inclusion in a magazine, newspaper, or broadcast.

Library of Congress Cataloging-in-Publication Data

Davison, Todd.
    Life after psychotherapy / by Todd Davison.
    p. cm.
    Includes bibliographical references and index.
    ISBN 1-56821-849-4 (alk. paper)
    1. Mental health. 2. Self-care, Health. 3. Psychotherapy.
    4. Psychotherapy—Termination. I. Title.
RA790.D397   1997
616.89—dc21   96-47407

Printed in the United States of America on acid-free paper. Jason Aronson Inc. offers books and cassettes. For information and catalog write to Jason Aronson Inc., 230 Livingston Street, Northvale, New Jersey 07647-1731. Or visit our website: http://www.aronson.com

Contents

Preface ix

Acknowledgments xi

Introduction xiii

Part I: The Return of Symptoms — 1

Depression — 4
    Sadness — 4
    Sleep disturbance — 5
    Appetite disturbance — 6
    Loss of energy — 6
    Loss of optimism and low self-esteem — 7
Anxiety — 9
Somatoform and Somatization Disorders — 11
Habit Disorders — 12
    What to do? — 13

Part II: Meditation Practice — 17

Sitting Meditation: Following Your Breath — 17
    Intrusive thoughts — 23
    A second strategy for intrusive thoughts — 24

Strong emotions ... 24
Anger at yourself ... 24
Bodily sensations ... 25
The impulse to act ... 26
Noises ... 27
Intruders ... 27
Times when sitting is not relaxing ... 27
Adding the lesson to breath awareness ... 28
Ending the meditation ... 28
Knowing when you are meditating the right way ... 28
Knowing you are meditating for the
    right length of time ... 28
Experiencing insights in meditation ... 29
Advanced Practice of Insight Meditation ... 29

Part III: Strategies for Healing Symptoms   33

Healing Depression ... 35
  Daily Practice for Depression ... 38
    Depression is my teacher. ... 39
    Depression is anger turned on myself. ... 39
    Angry feelings begin my healing journey. ... 41
    Forgiveness paves the road to peace of mind. ... 41
    I am never angry at the person I think. ... 43
    Whoever suffers is not me. ... 44
    All emotions are either love or fear. ... 45
    Oneness is the optimal view. ... 46
Healing Anxiety ... 47
  Daily Practice for Healing Anxiety ... 54
    Anxiety begins my healing journey. ... 55
    I do not know what distresses me. ... 55
    My stressors are grievances in my mind. ... 56
    I can feel peace instead of conflict. ... 57
    Forgiveness paves the road to peace of mind. ... 58
    I have projected the world I see. ... 59
    Oneness is the optimal view. ... 60

Healing Pain and Worries about My Body ... 61
   I will search my body as a window to my mind. ... 62
   My stressors are grievances in my mind. ... 65
   Angry feelings begin my healing journey. ... 66
   Forgiveness paves the road to peace of mind. ... 67
   Oneness is the optimal view. ... 68
Healing Habit Disorders ... 69
   My cravings are a window to my mind. ... 72
   Angry feelings begin my healing journey. ... 73
   Forgiveness paves the road to peace of mind. ... 73
   Oneness is the optimal view. ... 74
Options for Psychological and Pharmacological Interventions ... 75

Part IV: A Protective Maintenance Program ... 77

Establishing a Practice Routine ... 77
   Level 1: Reading and looking at your card during the day ... 78
   Level 2: Meditation plus level 1 ... 78
   Level 3: Write an example of using the day's lesson plus level 2 ... 81
   Level 4: Journaling in your *Disruptions, Dreams and Dilemmas* notebook plus level 3 ... 82
Goals of Psychotherapy ... 88
   1. Things are not the way I see them now. ... 89
   2. I am never emotional for the reasons I think because my childhood story distorts my adult perspective. ... 93
   3. Scripts for others are a part of my childhood story. ... 99
   4. Attachments are part of my childhood story. ... 102
   5. My sexual drives are a part of me. ... 104
   6. Aggressive drives are a part of me. ... 107
   7. Emotions are triggered by either love or fear. ... 109

8. Love is the answer.	117
9. Listening is love in action.	120
10. Oneness is an essential point of view.	123
11. Peace of mind is my only goal.	126
12. I will find no value in holding on to blame or guilt.	128
13. Forgiveness paves the road to peace of mind.	131
14. Now is the only time there is.	136
15. Healing is my choice to make.	139
16. Learning is a key to peace of mind and teaching is a good way to learn.	143
17. Laughter is the best medicine.	145
18. Today I will extend myself in kindness.	146
19. Today I will speak from a compassionate heart.	148
20. Search out the good and praise it.	150
21. I have an inner guide, the force, which I can access in quiet moments.	152
Frequently Asked Questions	156

Part V: Keeping It Going   161

Listening with Your Significant Other	161
Forming a Study Group	162
Other Resources	162
Finding Your Own Path	163
Continuing Study	163
Postscript	165

Index   167

Preface

Psychotherapy gives us an opportunity to develop emotional articulateness. It helps us become more neutral observers, less condemning toward our thoughts, fantasies, and emotions. It helps us learn how to observe our mental contents. Psychotherapy helps us see the myriad choices we have for any action, when before psychotherapy we could see but few. But if we do not practice these observing and choosing skills after therapy, they atrophy. Few psychotherapies teach us how to continue practicing (once treatment is ended) the observing and choosing functions that we learned with such great effort.

Psychoanalysts fare a little better. Psychoanalytic institutes provide a setting for lifelong study, practice, discussion, and teaching. Some attention is given to self-analysis even though very little is said about how that actually works. If we who have enjoyed the benefits of psychotherapy do not develop avenues for study, practice, discussion, and teaching after psychotherapy, then emotional articulateness, keen emotional observations, and a less condemning attitude toward thoughts and emotions will not be fully actualized. We will forget about stepping back from our intense emotions and looking for their contributions from childhood. Moreover, when action is necessary, we will not remember how many choices are available to us.

In this book we will consider a program of study, discussion, and formal practice of self-analysis and teaching in our life after psychotherapy.

Many of us waste significant portions of our lives trying to change others. Not only does this do little to endear us to the object of our attention but it ensures us an internal life of frustration. Others cannot be changed by our efforts, but we do have the power to change ourselves. Many of us choose to change ourselves through psychotherapy or psychoanalysis. As helpful as those changes are, they need constant maintenance. Just like any treasured relationship a relationship with ourselves requires time and effort. We can recapture the changes we once enjoyed from our psychotherapy by a daily program of study, discussion, practice, and teaching. This book outlines a program you can use to recapture the momentum of psychotherapy in your life.

Take thirty minutes each morning and you will change your relationship to your thoughts and feelings. You will change from a person who is compelled by your thoughts and feelings to a person who is a calm witness to these internal events. Catastrophe will disappear and give way to challenge. Anxiety will disappear and give way to energy. Depression will evaporate and transform to moments of blame forgiven. Shame will disappear and become errors to be corrected. These shifts in perception can begin today if you choose to make them. It is your life. It is your choice. Take a chance. Just do it!

Acknowledgments

Thanks to Carolyn Washburne, Christine Nuernberg, and Ruth Holst who edited this book. Also, thanks to Renée, my wife, who helped me think of examples for many of the lessons. Thanks to Barbara Klemans, my sister, who is an ongoing source of support and ideas. Thanks to Susan Deutsch, my office manager, who is one of the best psychotherapists I know. Thanks to all my colleagues at Columbia Hospital who support this work including Wayne Boulanger, M.D., our chief of staff, who is one of the best writers I know; Gayle Mendeloff, M.D., a fine surgeon and our upcoming chief of staff; Lyle Henry, M.D., a pioneer in the field of minimally invasive surgery; David Shapiro, M.D., a gifted internist and an excellent meditation teacher; Steve Robbins, M.D., an expert spinal surgeon, who lets me collaborate with him in helping patients with back pain; Jim Stoll, M.D., a fine spinal surgeon; Dick Fritz, M.D., a superb oncologist and hematologist who is a true supporter of mind–body medicine; Jack Chamberlain, M.D., who has become so proficient at meditation that he is sought as a teacher; Gholi Darien, M.D., a special friend and a fine internist gifted in understanding the psychology of his patients; Jim Volberding, M.D., the Sherlock Holmes of internists; Andy Seter, M.D., an occupational medicine specialist par excellence; Gerald McCarthy, M.D., our vice-president of medical affairs and one of the only people I know who is equally adept in medicine and management; Sister Renée Rose, Chairman of the Board of Columbia-St. Mary's Inc. and a true supporter of mind–body medicine; Doug Klink, M.D., a fine endocrinologist and friend; Bruce Wilson, M.D., a cardiologist with heart; Scott Stanwyck, M.D., an orthopedist who knows the knee like no other; Jed Vitamvas, M.D., an ob-gyn with a special gift for empathy; Ed Dunn, M.D., a gifted cardiac surgeon who has helped us in many ways; Rich Staudacher, M.D., a cardiologist and supporter of mind–body medicine; Harry Prosen, M.D., the boss; Brent Field, M.D., a gifted internist; Jeff Taxman, M.D., my partner; Paul Westrick, a new-found helper in mind–body medicine, and a special thanks to the person who makes all the mind–body programs possible at Columbia, John Schuler, President and Chief Executive Officer at Columbia-St. Mary's Inc.

A special thanks to Joan Metzler, manager of Behavioral Medicine. Thanks to Terry Koch, Colleen Flores, JoAnn Hankwitz, Jo Sims, Kate Rouse, and Sunny Mendeloff, the therapists who implement our programs and Renée Kueler, our persistent program assistant. Thanks to Tom Kopka, Jim Chamberlain, and Tom Ryan, our HealthQuest instructors. Thanks to all the nurses who use these programs throughout Columbia Hospital, especially Joann Timmerman, who uses these techniques every day with our patients in the day hospital program, and Caryl Zaar, our stellar nurse-manager and facilitator. Thanks to our star facilitators for attitudinal healing, John Puestow, Betty Gaedke, and David Clowers. A very special thanks to Peg Mayer who has been my nutrition counselor for the past five years—what patience!

Introduction

How many of us have had this experience? Some time after completing a successful psychotherapy, we find ourselves immersed in symptoms of anxiety and depression. The same symptoms that brought us to treatment have returned and we do not have a clue as to why. We expected the therapeutic gain from psychotherapy to last forever, but it slipped away from us. What do we do now?

These were the questions that drove me to look for a method to extend the gains made in individual psychotherapy and to bring life back to the process. First I needed to find a method for introspection. A colleague, Tom Kopka, suggested meditation, and after trying it with his guidance I found it to be the perfect way to continue looking below the surface of my urgent thoughts and feelings. Another colleague, Jim Boeglin, suggested journaling. The two, meditation and journaling, worked better together than either one worked alone. They provided avenues for practice and expression. So I set forth with a method. Then I needed to find some goals. A third colleague, Jann McClintock, suggested I read *A Course in Miracles*®. This remarkable book is an encyclopedia of psychoanalytic goals. Putting the goals of *A Course in Miracles*® together with meditation and journaling is Attitudinal Healing, an enterprise started by Gerald Jampolsky, M.D., who personally helped me begin our program at Columbia Hospital in Milwaukee. The program gave an opportunity for introspection, discussion, study, and teaching. Those four components are crucial to moving beyond psychotherapy to self-care and self-guidance.

I am lucky to have found a way to extend my psychotherapy into a process by which I can help myself. Some of us are not so fortunate as to have mental health professionals around who will try to help us.

Phil was 37 years old. He was doing well in his business; his workers admired him, and he was fond of them. His family was thriving and he was popular in his social circle. He lived life with a balanced sense of moderation. He loved his wife and she loved him. His 5-year-old daughter, Andria, thought he was the greatest. His son, Phil Jr., was an honor student in junior high school and an extraordinary soccer player. Yet Phil was extremely unhappy. As he sat on the side of his bed thinking about suicide, he asked himself what had gone wrong. Two years before he had completed four years of intensive psychotherapy with a respected psychoanalyst whom he had come to appreciate and value. For two years his life had had its ups and downs but overall he dealt with the problems with wisdom and wit. Now, however, he felt tired, hopeless, and miserable, and he had no idea why.

Janis was a 52-year-old mother of two grown children when her husband divorced her for a younger woman. When he left, she seemed to forget everything she had learned in psychoanalysis, which she had completed seven years before. She took every opportunity to deride her ex-husband to her two grown daughters, who felt burdened and torn by her complaints. One day she was attempting to shop at a neighborhood drugstore when she became short of breath, dizzy, and faint. She was rushed to the hospital for a suspected heart attack, but all her cardiac studies were normal. They had also been normal the other three times she had been rushed to the hospital in the last two weeks.

Bob drove a bus for a living. He was late for work every day for two weeks because he felt he had to check the locks on the doors twenty times before he could leave the house. Five years before, when he stopped his psychotherapy, and for the next four and a half years, he was fine but now he was experiencing a return of symptoms stronger than when he had entered psychotherapy.

Father John had a successful life as a priest and a psychotherapist, and had finished psychoanalysis twelve years before he was revisited by symptoms. He hated his work and he hated himself despite the recent success of a book he had written on spirituality and psychotherapy. He was bothered by nagging back pain and muscle aches in different parts of his body. He had diarrhea several times a week. His doctors could find no signs of pathology in his back or in his gastrointestinal tract after doing all the sophisticated imaging studies, including MRIs, CT scans, and colonoscopic examinations. They diagnosed him as having fibromyalgia and an irritable bowel syndrome.

Belinda finished a successful psychotherapy three years before she began overeating, overdrinking, and smoking again. She knew that she had addressed these problems in psychotherapy. She knew they were symptoms of other hungers but in experiencing the return of these symptoms she felt out of control. She wanted to be able to deal with the problems on her own but did not know where to start.

These former psychotherapy patients had something in common. After psychotherapy ended they paid only modest attention to keeping the fire of introspection alive in their lives. They had little opportunity for study, discussion, and teaching of an ongoing life philosophy. They treated psychotherapy as one might treat getting a car fixed. You get the car fixed until it breaks again. But even cars get the oil changed and an occasional tune-up. They did not treat themselves that well. They did not have a protective maintenance program. They all learned by a circuitous route that they needed a better plan. I had just begun a plan for myself when I met this group of patients. I had begun to feel anxious without knowing why. I had not made time for myself until I started my program. We met in a group to bring a new plan to life. This book contains what we discovered to bring us new life beyond psychotherapy. Before I explain the plan, let us look at where we had gone wrong.

We had failed to recognize the onset of depression, anxiety, and somatic symptoms in our lives and did not turn for help until a crisis forced us to do so. A better way to proceed is to begin, from early in therapy, a practice routine that you can use for the rest of your life. If you did not do that in your own psychotherapy, the time to start your protective maintenance program is now. In this book I will discuss a program that you can begin today and continue for the rest of your life to make your life after psychotherapy one filled with peace of mind.

But what happened to our peace of mind? What we forgot is that forgetting is relentless. Repression, the means of forgetting, is an ever-present danger. Freud said that the mind is like a jungle. We make a clearing in our battle to make the unconscious conscious, but our gains are only temporary. The plant life in the jungle swallows up our insights if we do not constantly maintain our hard-won foothold in the path of the relentless force of repression. It is normal to forget unpleasant memories but it is just as normal to forget skills that we do not use every day. While forgetting unpleasant memories is not so bad, as long as they are not deeply repressed and can be remembered with a shift in our attention, forgetting to stand back and observe our minds when we are in the throes of urgent emotional reactions is not so useful. However, it is a natural consequence of not practicing, not continuing our learning, not discussing, and not teaching. We forgot that the skills we had learned in observing our thoughts and feelings would dwindle without practice. When we were in intensive psychotherapy we practiced several times a week and we and our therapist formed an enthusiastic group. We studied. We were teachers to each other.

The part of psychotherapy that is often emphasized is the cognitive part. We think of what we learned about competition and revenge, sexual attraction, and fantasies. We forget that another aspect of what we learned is to be observant of these mental contents without judging them. Without practice, our abilities to witness mental content withers like a plant without sunshine or dies like a fish without water.

If we worked hard in our psychotherapy, we learned a few important lessons, including that our perceptions are frequently distorted by our past and that human perception is quite limited. We learned that we have two basic emotions: love and fear. We learned to heal ourselves by taking time to look deeply into the causes of our impulses and emotions and to rebuke and then forgive those who offend us, in our mind rather than in action. We learned that a constant effort to learn about how our mind works is a prerequisite for maintaining our peace of mind. And we learned to trust ourselves after introspection. What we may not have learned was how to practice daily what we had learned in order to maintain our clearing in the jungle. The best way to learn is to keep ourselves open to inspiration no matter where or when it comes and to teach what we have learned by example.

During a break at The American Psychoanalytic Association committee meetings recently, a group of us, all senior training analysts from psychoanalytic institutes around the country, went to lunch. I asked a friend of mine, Larry Inderbitzen, from Atlanta, who I knew had had a bout with high blood pressure several years before, how his blood pressure was. He said that it was fine now. I asked what medication he was on, and he said that he was on no medication. I asked how he managed to do that and he said, "meditation." All eyes turned toward him. Gradually, one by one, several members of the group admitted meditating daily. It seemed that we all had come to the same conclusion. You cannot keep the fires of introspection alive in your life without daily practice. To do this many of us had chosen the route of daily meditation.

Larry's story got even better. His physicians were skeptical. They did not believe that he could control his hypertension by meditation alone, so they put him on 24-hour telemetric blood pressure monitoring. Not only was his blood pressure under perfect control, but the times it was lowest was when he was meditating and *when he was conducting psychoanalysis*. Now stop to think about that for a moment. If there is any time in one's life when one is focused in the moment it is when meditating, because in meditation we focus all our energy on maintaining a moment-to-moment awareness of the present. The same is true for the psychoanalyst or psychotherapist who is listening intently for the moment-to-moment shifts in his client's associations and affects. And the same goes for the client in psychoanalysis or psychotherapy who is attempting to develop a part of herself that is constantly observing the present moment without judging the thoughts and feelings that emerge. The endeavors of working as an analyst, therapist, client, and mindfulness meditation practitioner focus on living in the present moment and living there to the fullest. So it occurred to me that meditation may be the optimal setting for keeping self-analysis or self-psychotherapy alive in my life.

I tried it for myself. I got a few friends to try it with me. Then I got some of my clients to try it too. We all agreed that meditation plus a few clear goals was a splendid protective maintenance program.

Mindfulness meditation is the simplest form of meditation. It does not attempt to create a blank mind. It attempts to create an observing part of our mind that can look at all our thoughts and feelings without judging, just like we did in psychoanalysis and psychotherapy. Unlike psychotherapy, we do not attempt to put these thoughts and feelings into words. Having a successful period of time in psychotherapy is a great aid for the meditation practitioner because we already have the words to fit the concepts that leap into our minds. Mindfulness meditation attempts to help us get in touch with the two most important and deepest parts of our being: the observer and the chooser. By noticing what is on our minds and continuously choosing to redirect our attention to our breath we reinforce those two crucial mental functions of observing and choosing. We learn to step back from our impulses and our reflexive actions to find that these too can be observed, and when we observe them, we have choices that we did not know were there before our mindfulness training.

What I hope to impart to you in this book is a way to begin meditation practice that will allow you to relax, use your psychotherapeutic articulateness to the fullest, and be at peace in the present.

This book is divided into five parts: first, we will examine the signs of forgetting, the return of symptoms; second, we will learn a form of meditation practice; third, we will address strategies for healing when symptoms reappear; fourth, we will examine a protective maintenance program; and fifth, we will discuss keeping our program going.

Part I: The Return of Symptoms

There are any number of psychiatric symptoms but the most recurrent ones are the ones we will discuss here. The most frequently disturbing psychiatric symptoms are those of depression, anxiety, somatic aches and pains, and habit disorders such as overeating, overdrinking, and oversmoking. By far the most troubling of these is depression. It is estimated that as many as one person in ten has disabling symptoms of depression at some time in life, and everyone has some symptoms of depression at times. There may be no more debilitating condition than depression and for that reason we will begin our discussion with it. In practice we can assume that all symptoms—depression, anxiety, somatic ones, and habit disorders begin with angry feelings that are not dealt with in an effective way. The angry feelings are a reaction to fear that some cherished desire will not be gratified. The cherished desire often comes more from some childhood belief than a realistic adult assessment.

Here is the way it works. John entered his office after a vacation to find that he had been moved from the office adjoining his boss's to a big office with windows down the hall. He was immediately furious. He knew that it would not be politic to go ranting down the hallway, cursing the gods, so he pushed down his angry feelings. He became a little anxious that he might spout off in some way that would alienate him from his boss, so he put a smile on his face and calmly knocked on his boss's door. Greg, his boss and mentor, answered the door smiling broadly.

"Surprise! How does it feel to finally have a decent-sized office with windows?" Greg asked.

John knew now that he was not being punished but rewarded. How could he have been so angry with Greg?

"Great, just great! Thank you very much."

As the weeks passed John felt more and more isolated from Greg. They no longer met at the water cooler. They no longer got each other coffee. They no longer shared sidewalk consultations as frequently as they had before. John was angry at Greg but he did not let himself experience those feelings. Each time he did, he felt a little nervous, and then the angry feelings went away.

John slept restlessly at night. He became worried about the performance of his pension plan. He was irritable with his children. Why did the kids take so long to finish their homework? Why did Jane fix the same old meals night after night? John felt afraid that the plane might crash when he was scheduled to fly on a business trip. He lost his appetite and he lost weight. He became worried that he had cancer. He had a headache that just would not go away. Maybe he had cancer that had metastasized to the brain. He hated himself for being so thoughtless of his family and of Greg. He could not be readily awakened in the morning. He had no energy. He drank too much and he started smoking his pipe even when he did not want to smoke. He thought about ending it all. He was depressed.

That is the way symptoms happen in real life. First strong angry feelings are suppressed. Then when the anger tends to rise to the surface, we feel nervous and try to push it down. That is the symptom of anxiety. We worry about our bodily aches and pains. We eat too much, drink too much, and smoke too much as actions designed to give substitute gratification and push our anger and fear out of mind. We get angry at ourselves for oral excesses. We worry about weight gain and what it will do to our blood pressure. We worry about catastrophic illness. That is somatization. Finally, we are depleted and we hate ourselves for just the thing that we were reluctant to feel angry at someone else about in the beginning. John was reluctant to feel angry at Greg for being so thoughtless as not to recognize that John's attachment to him was so great that no window or big office could replace the closeness they shared with adjoining offices. But instead of feeling at ease with those angry feelings toward Greg and working them out, he tried to push them out of mind and ended up blaming himself for his own thoughtlessness, which was just what he was reluctant to feel angry at Greg about. He felt a loss of self-esteem and hated himself for being weak.

Had John been in psychotherapy at the time or had he been meditating he might have discovered that what occurred between Greg and him recapitulated the feelings he had toward his mother and father when his little sister was born. When she was born, John was moved out of the windowless bedroom adjoining his parents' bedroom.

A big deal was made of his great big new bedroom at the end of the hall with all its windows that let him see outside. He was not consoled. He moped around the way he had seen his father mope when his mother did not do his father's bidding.

Even though depression is the endpoint of the symptom train and a depletion syndrome as opposed to the anxiety that often precedes it, we will begin with depression rather than anxiety because it is a more debilitating symptom.

DEPRESSION

Depression is a set of symptoms, including sadness that lingers, sleep disturbance, appetite disturbance, loss of energy, loss of optimism, and a low self-esteem. When a person is depressed he feels helpless and hopeless. Let us examine each one of these in more detail.

Sadness

Sadness is a feeling of loss. Something or someone is gone and there is no bringing that person or opportunity back. When we are sad we feel on the verge of tears. We feel emptiness. We feel a gnawing in the pit of our stomachs.

Sadness is normal and it is especially normal in grief. In grief we acknowledge the loss of someone important in our life. In grief, sadness is time limited. When we lose a loved one, the sadness is greatest at first and then it fades over a period of months. If we allow ourselves to feel loss without hating ourselves for it and without expecting ourselves to have as much energy as we normally do, then the sadness fades with time. If we hate ourselves for our grief, we become depressed. This form of depression is called *pathological grief*.

Sleep disturbance

Sleep disturbance can be either sleeping too much or too little. The most common form of sleep disturbance is difficulty falling asleep. That often suggests that we have worries in our lives that we are not addressing. The second most common form is early morning awakening. That usually means that there is something bothering us that we can escape for periods of time in sleep that we have not faced adequately. The third form is frequent awakening with difficulty falling back to sleep. The fourth form is difficulty falling asleep, frequent awakening during the night with trouble falling back asleep, plus early morning awakening with a desperate feeling of not being rested or not having slept at all. This is the most disturbing of all sleep disorders and the one most closely associated with severe depression. Another form of sleep disturbance associated with depression is sleeping too much and awakening feeling unrested.

None of these forms of sleep disturbance is by itself an indication of depression. Other illnesses, such as hyper- or hypothyroidism, metabolic and endocrine disorders, cardiovascular disorders, alcohol and other drug use, and primary sleep disorders such as sleep apnea can cause sleep disturbance. Anyone with a sleep disturbance should have a thorough history and physical examination by his internist or family medicine practitioner.

Appetite disturbance

Loss of appetite most commonly accompanies depression. In more severe depressions weight loss accompanies appetite disturbance. In some depressions the opposite happens and the individual experiences an increased appetite, compulsive eating, and weight gain. A common form of depression which is paradoxically called *atypical depression* is one in which the patient has increased appetite, gains weight, and sleeps too much.

Appetite increase or decrease is not only a sign of depression so it is incumbent upon anyone suffering an appetite change to first have a thorough physical examination before trying psychotherapy, psychopharmacology, or self-help. Gastrointestinal illness can affect appetite, as can almost any physical disorder.

Loss of energy

Most people who are depressed feel a loss of energy, but not all. Some are so frightened by a loss of energy that they overcompensate by becoming excessively energetic. But most depressed patients just have no energy, no get-up-and-go. They would like to sleep but only are able to toss and turn.

Loss of energy can be primarily metabolic in origin. A patient was referred to me for symptoms of increased energy and elation, most commonly found in hypomanic states or hyperthyroidism. The patient, a teacher in his early fifties, had become overly talkative and outgoing at work. His adoring students and fellow faculty members knew that he was acting totally out of character. I saw him once and thought the same thing. He was staying up all night working on great ideas, calling all over the world just to keep in touch with old friends, and teaching exercise classes in the time that he normally reserved for resting. I was about to start him on lithium, a mood stabilizer, when I looked at his laboratory data and noticed that his TSH, an indicator of thyroid function, had not been reported from the laboratory. When I called the lab they reported a very high TSH, indicating low thyroid functioning. He was so afraid of decreased energy, which he associated with the death of his father, that he pushed himself to excessive activity rather than give in to the loss of energy that he felt in his quiet moments. Adjustment of his thyroid and short-term psychotherapy were all he needed to return to normal.

Most depressed patients feel tired all the time, even when they first awaken in the morning. Some feel especially tired in the morning but seem to rally when the sun goes down. They hate to go to sleep, because they know that another terrible morning awaits them. Others feel fine in the morning but fatigue in the afternoon. A few depressed patients feel fine when they awaken but a few hours later they are completely drained. Most depressed patients feel one form of decreased energy or another.

Loss of optimism and low self-esteem

Most depressed patients feel that life is awful: it has always been awful and it will always be awful. If you ask them how long they have felt this way they will say "forever." If you ask someone who knows them well the same question, their loved one is likely to report, "John was upbeat until he accidentally ran over our dog with the car last June. He hasn't been himself since then." If you ask John about that, he might disagree and insist that he has always felt bad and running over the dog had nothing to do with it.

A part of the loss of optimism is a tendency to blame. If I feel terrible, there must be someone to blame. Sometimes the blame will be aimed at others but it will ultimately be turned back on myself. With the blame turned back on myself I feel low self-esteem and self-hatred. It is good to note this blaming tendency because it is in dealing with blame that the psychological treatment of depression begins.

As with the other symptoms of depression, loss of optimism not only indicates depression, it can be the sign of a more traditional physical disorder, so a complete physical examination is in order. But barring a major cardiovascular, endocrine, metabolic, or other physical disorder, a primary depression is likely. Not all depressions are severe or clinically debilitating. Sometimes mild depressions are self-limiting. Mild depressions are normal and may even be useful.

Everyone feels depressed at times. Depression can be seen as a normal condition, a warning signal that it is time to rethink priorities and to reset our goals. If we use moments of depression as an indicator that it is time to do some maintenance work on our minds and on our lives, then depression is normal and useful. But depression unchecked can also be a dark hole that we cannot climb out of without outside help. Later we will consider a series of exercises designed to stop depression before it becomes such a hole but first let us consider the second group of symptoms most likely to give us trouble: anxiety.

ANXIETY

In our story about John and Greg, remember that anxiety was stirred up to get John to push down his angry feelings. That is what anxiety does. Underneath anxiety is an angry feeling we do not wish to face. And under that is the fear that some cherished desire will go unfulfilled. That cherished desire may have more to do with a childhood belief than any adult need.

Anxiety is a complex of feelings including hypervigilance, dread, and fear associated with something known or unknown in the future. The smallest degree of anxiety is called *signal anxiety*. Signal anxiety is such a small quantity of fear that we often do not even register it consciously. An example of signal anxiety is when the stoplight turns green and we hesitate for a moment before accelerating. During that moment's hesitation we glance right and left just to make sure that intersecting traffic has come to a stop. Where is the anger in that, you may ask? The anger suppressed is the irritation that we have to stop for something. In signal anxiety we may not feel a sense of caution for more than a split second. If that cautionary impulse were magnified we might sit there in a panic, our heart and breathing racing, numbness around our mouth, the experience of a full-blown panic attack.

Anxiety disorders come in various packages. If a person feels anxiety a lot of the time with two or more general topics of worry we label this a *generalized anxiety disorder*. If the anxiety comes on as an attack out of the blue, lasts twenty minutes and goes away, we call that a *panic attack*. If those panic attacks come on most frequently when a person leaves his house so that he avoids leaving his house altogether, we call that *panic attacks with agoraphobia*.

Then there are the varieties of anxiety disorders that lead to more circumscribed forms of avoidance. A *phobia* is a powerful need or desire to avoid something due to exaggerated fear. Some individuals fear falling, so they avoid high places and flying. Some people fear being closed in, so they avoid elevators and small rooms. Some fear spiders, so they avoid places where they are more likely to see spiders. There are many other forms of phobia, including a phobic lifestyle where one must keep moving all the time to avoid sitting down and facing feelings.

Another form of anxiety disorder called *obsessive compulsive disorder* requires a person to repeatedly check things such as making sure the stove is turned off twenty times before he can go to sleep or checking to see that all the doors are locked before she can sit down to read. An obsessive concern may erupt and the person may become worried about her health or fearful of some other catastrophe that she cannot get out of her mind. This form of anxiety disorder may include a fear of germs leading to a person's washing his hands fifty times a day or scrubbing the walls and cabinets in the kitchen until they are damaged. If the person at the green light had to check right and left twenty times before he could accelerate, that, too, would be part of an obsessive-compulsive anxiety disorder.

Anxiety is often a useful warning that protects us from rushing into potentially dangerous situations. In anxiety disorders this normal emotion is magnified in situations where little objective cause for fear exists.

In the forms just outlined, I have never seen a person who was not able to come to grips with the sources of his discomfort and to face them. Anxiety and depression can be a gift because they may be viewed as beacons that light the way to areas in our mental life that require our attention. Most people with the outright symptoms of anxiety and depression can be helped or can help themselves. But there is a more difficult group of symptoms called *somatoform* or *somatization disorders* that seem like simple physical complaints but really disguise unrecognized anxiety and anger.

SOMATOFORM AND SOMATIZATION DISORDERS

A person with a somatoform or somatization disorder does not recognize that he is depressed, anxious, and angry. If a physician suggests as much, such a patient is likely to speak to the doctor with indignation and hostility: "I wonder if you would say that if you had diarrhea three times a week and if your back hurt so much you could not sit for more than five minutes at a time. How would you feel if every muscle in your body was sore to touch?" Rather than alienate their patients, some physicians treat them with analgesics and other medications to address their symptoms. They listen to their complaints and readjust their medications. Some of these patients become severely depressed when their anger comes to the surface and they turn it back on themselves rather than permit the angry feelings. Some physicians treating these patients symptomatically use higher doses of a multiplicity of drugs. If the physician recognizes an underlying depression he may begin a relatively safe antidepressant, such as sertraline. When the obvious signs of depression clear, the somatic complaints lessen for a while but then return if the psychology of the patient cannot be addressed.

By far the most prevalent of these disorders is tension back pain. In his book *Healing Back Pain*,[1] John Sarno, M.D., suggests that as many as 80 percent of the population has a history of pain syndromes. He states that back and neck pain are the number one cause of worker absenteeism in the United States and he estimates that 56 billion dollars per year is spent on the treatment of these disorders. He also suggests that many other physical conditions receive significant emotional contributions, including peptic ulcer disease, indigestion, hiatal hernia, irritable bowel syndrome, hay fever, asthma, headaches, eczema, dizziness, ringing in the ears, and frequent urination.

HABIT DISORDERS

Habit disorders are symptoms that arise when we are frustrated that we are not getting the gratification we want. We turn to immediate fixes to reduce our frustration. Eating, drinking, and smoking are among the most common habit disorders. The most frequent ways of dealing with these excesses is to try by willpower to overcome them. We diet instead of eat. We abstain from alcohol instead of drinking too much. We stop smoking instead of enjoying an occasional smoke. In other words we substitute a resolute denial for our excesses. But compulsive abstention does not address the underlying frustration at not getting the gratification that we long for.

---

1. John E. Sarno. (1991). *Healing Back Pain*. New York: Warner Books.

Are these symptoms a curse or a gift? I think of symptoms as a gift from our body to us. Our body is telling us that we have some work to do in the emotional maintenance department. We can learn to recognize these symptoms as signs to begin our self-help work.

What to do?

We all have these symptoms at some time in our lives. We will look at specific strategies to deal with each of these symptom clusters in Part III of this book. Anyone who has been in psychotherapy may recognize times in her life when she has been troubled by one or a combination of these symptom clusters. When we get bogged down in depression, anxiety, somatic concerns, or disordered habits, there are some clear things to do and a clear order in which to do them:

1. Get a physical examination from a doctor you trust. If medical treatment is warranted, follow the medical regimen. That regimen may include the use of a new broad spectrum form of antidepressant and antianxiety medication called selective serotonin re-uptake inhibitors (SSRIs) such as sertraline, fluoxetine, and paroxetine. I favor sertraline as the first line of these medications. I have heard colleagues say that if we remove the symptoms with medications we may rob the individual of motivation for psychotherapy. That has not been my experience. When prescribing sertraline, for example, I suggest to my patient that he can expect a 15 percent reduction in his symptoms of anxiety and depression. This symptom reduction may be viewed

as an opportunity for new learning that may enable him to stop taking this medication in the future.
2. When your symptoms of depression, anxiety, or somatic complaints reach a level that permits you the energy to work on them, turn to a psychotherapist you trust.
3. If you are working with a psychotherapist use these self-help suggestions in conjunction with your treatment.
4. If you use these self-help suggestions be prepared to use them indefinitely. You must become your own psychotherapist and, as with any profession, you have to practice to stay proficient in your field. Think of psychotherapy as learning to fly your life in a Link Trainer, the mock-up of an airplane that pilots use to familiarize themselves with a real airplane. Later you get into the actual life and fly solo. And finally you become proficient and become an instructor. So be ready to begin a self-help practice regimen that you will continue several times a week for the rest of your life. You will look forward to your practice as it enhances your moment-to-moment life experience.

In the rest of this book we will examine strategies for dealing with depression, anxiety, somatization, and habit disorders. Most of us have a combination of all of these, even though one form of symptom may predominate at one time and a different symptom at another. In moderation, all these symptoms are good. Depression is good because it is an early warning signal to reassess our priorities. Anxiety is good because it tells us that we are experiencing danger. Somatic symptoms are good because they lead us to remember childhood experiences that affect our adult life. Habit disorders are good because they are warning signs to look inward and see why we are not getting what we want from life. Physical sensations encode emotions and memories. They are the storehouse of important life memories that we can get in touch with by meditation practice. Physical symptoms also remind us to keep our bodies in the best shape we can. So it is useful to learn a practice that addresses all these symptoms every day.

First we will examine meditation practice. Then we will look at the strategies for addressing different symptoms separately. Then we will combine them, and finally we will examine preventive medicine approaches to beating the blues in our life beyond psychotherapy.

Part II:
Meditation Practice

**SITTING MEDITATION:
FOLLOWING YOUR BREATH**

One of the most important skills you can learn in order to fly solo in your psychotherapy is how to meditate. One of my colleagues, Mary Jo Sims, M.S.N., a clinical nurse practitioner and a person whose judgment I trust, keeps asking me to think of another word for this. She says, "Meditation sounds too much like religious practice." I have tried, but relaxation exercise misses the whole point. Relaxation is a part of meditation but it is not the most important part and no other word conveys that part very well. The most important part of meditation is the observing part. And that is the part that is most like what we learn to do in psychotherapy and psychoanalysis. We learn to observe our thoughts and emotions as thoughts and emotions rather than as being our totality. They are just a part of us and a part that we can observe without acting on it. That is the lesson we forget most quickly when we stop our psychotherapy. We tend to become embroiled in our emotions as if they were our whole self and as if we had to act on them. As we become better at observing we are able to see choices we did not know we had. Choosing is the second most important practice in meditation. We practice choosing each time we decide to redirect our attention back to our breath. There are many ways to achieve a relaxed, observing stance but the one I like best is following the breath.

Following your breath is one of the most useful forms of sitting meditation practice. In following your breath you sit quietly with your eyes closed or slightly open and focused a few feet in front of you, in a comfortable, erect posture. You breathe through your nose, if that is comfortable for you. Let your abdomen rise with the in-breath and fall with the out-breath. Think "In" with your in-breath and "Out" with your out-breath or just be aware of your breath as it comes in and out of your body. Our breath is our most important form of nourishment and the one from which we can least abstain. Tom Ryan, a colleague of mine, told me that we can live forty-nine days without food, seven days without water, and only seven minutes without breath. So paying attention to our breath is like honoring a fine meal or a cool sip of water.

When we follow our breath other thoughts intrude; *observe* them without judging, then gently *choose* to move your attention back to your abdomen as it moves in and out with your breath. Following your breath is following the rise and fall of your abdomen or following the sense of breath at your nostrils. In each sequence you observe and you choose. Every moment you are exercising these two most important mental functions. You are practicing them and you are convincing yourself that you can observe any thought, feeling, or fantasy while exercising the choice to be at peace with it rather than compelled to act on it or act to avoid it. This is a solitary form of the practice we once exercised in psychotherapy—observing—that is, observing and choosing to sit with our thoughts and feelings, but now we practice it with simple breath awareness.

Not everyone is comfortable with abdominal movement when breathing. If you are not, you can be aware of your breath at your nostrils. Notice the air move "in" through your nostrils with your in-breath and "out" across your nostrils with your out-breath.

Above all do not get hung up on doing it "right." Any way you do it is right. The whole idea of focusing on your breath is to teach you that you have a choice as to where to focus your observing mind. Any moment you wish to exercise that choice you can choose to focus back in the present on your breath, your primary nourishment on this planet. You become convinced that you can focus your observing instrument in the present without acting on mental content. So don't make a federal case out of it. It's not brain surgery. Don't use this as an opportunity to give yourself a hard time.

Remember, the purpose of meditation is NOT to create a blank mind. It is to change your relationship to your thoughts and feelings. The relationship change is from one with a sense of urgency to act to one with a sense of calm, observing nonjudgment that highlights your ability to choose what to observe and what to do.

Practice, in this context, simply means doing, as opposed to preparing for something or improving something.

Formal meditation means meditation done in a particular form, such as sitting, walking, exercising, yoga, or tai chi.

Meditation is useful because it slows all the systems in the body and gives us a chance to observe our minds and bodies. It gives us a chance to recognize the choices we have. Neurologically it opens synapses between the left prefrontal cortex and the limbic system, and the left prefrontal cortex and the right prefrontal cortex. The neurological effects of this practice permit us to witness our emotions without jumping into action prematurely, before choosing to act.

Meditation may serve as a platform from which to launch a lesson to practice each day. In the meditation we discuss here, there are two parts: the formal sitting meditation we encourage you to do each morning, and the minute-long meditation we encourage you to do several times each day around a particular lesson for the day. One way to combine a lesson with breathing during meditation is to think of the first half of the lesson on the in-breath and the second half of the lesson on the out-breath. IN, *"As for the future,"* OUT, *"I trust the force."* Repeat the process three to five times at the beginning of meditation. Then follow your breath. At the end of meditation, over three to five breath cycles, repeat the lesson again. Then several times during the day take a minute to repeat the lesson for the day.

Any length of time is useful for meditation, from one minute to one hour. Each person has a different optimal time. Try different times like five, ten, fifteen, twenty, and thirty minutes to find out which one is best for you. You will know when you find the optimal length of time because it will feel short. If the time feels long, meditate for a shorter period of time.

At first in formal meditation practice it is best to follow your breath rather than trying to imagine different things. As you breathe in, think to yourself, "In." As you breathe out, think, "Out." As you do this, other thoughts, emotions, and bodily sensations come to mind. As soon as you are aware of them, label them without judging, "Thought," "To do list," "Feeling." Then choose to return to your abdomen or nostrils, "In" and "Out." When you choose to refocus on your breath, do so with gentleness. Kindly and gently usher yourself back to your breath. Once you have experience in practicing sitting meditation, you may find that you can enter a relaxed state, fully aware of the present, with your eyes open, any time you choose.

After you become confident that you can return your attention to your breath any time you choose, if only for a few seconds, you may choose useful subjects of attention other than your breath, such as bodily sensations, thoughts, or emotions. Instead of returning to your breath as soon as you become aware of other subjects, you may choose to follow your bodily sensations, thoughts, and emotions simply by noticing them. When you face these sensations, thoughts, and emotions without judging them, without using them as planned action, and without being moved to act as they come to mind, you optimize formal meditation practice. By doing this, you learn to be at peace rather than scurrying around with a sense of urgency.

At times sitting is not comfortable for meditation; at those times lying, walking, or exercising may be used. When walking and exercising, you may choose to focus on a repetitive motion rather than the rise and fall of your abdomen or your breath through your nostrils. When walking or exercising, for example, you may count the number of right leg movements up to ten and then back down again. In between the calm moments, when you are counting, ideas will spring to mind that would not have come without a calm surface. Frequently, bursts of inspiration immediately follow meditation. A neighbor of mine, Dan Steininger, is an insurance company CEO. He says that after he meditates, he is ready to pick up his dictaphone and dictate six memos because all kinds of good ideas come to him following meditation. This is a common occurrence. When you quiet the surface of your mind you tap into deeper levels of intuition. After meditation you can process these intuitive ideas through your mature sense of reason, and bingo! Out pop some really creative ideas.

In all meditation practice the idea is to let the mind be still and calm in order to be able to observe more clearly. But no matter how peaceful we try to be, there are moments when it is very difficult to calm the mind. Then, additional measures can be useful. One of the most useful methods for calming a restless mind is soundlessly repeating a simple, two-syllable, nonsense word. Some people call this word a *mantra*. When following your breath is not calming, saying over and over to yourself "lapko" or any other two-syllable word may bring deeper peace by calming the nagging inner voices. Sometimes counting the out-breaths serves a similar purpose. Count the out-breaths up to ten and then back down again.

When you practice sitting meditation, sit still in an upright chair, in an erect posture with both feet on the floor. Close your eyes and focus on your breathing. Actually, focus on the rise and fall of your abdomen as you breathe. Breathe through your nose when that is comfortable for you. Feel the breath come in as your abdomen expands, and feel the breath flow out as your abdomen contracts. Sometimes when counting the out-breaths (1,

2, 3, 4, 5, up to 10 and then back down again), controlling the pace of your breathing to less than eight breaths per minute is useful. If thoughts drift into your mind, observe them without judging; then choose to focus back to noticing the rise and fall of your abdomen or your breath count. The act of being aware of your thoughts without judging them is to establish a nonjudging witness within yourself.

To manage sitting meditation effectively, you will need to learn how to handle all sorts of things: intrusive thoughts, strong emotions, anger at yourself, bodily sensations, the impulse to act, noises, intruders, times when sitting is not relaxing, adding the lesson for the day, ending the meditation, knowing when you are meditating the right way and for the right length of time, and experiencing insights in meditation. Now let us consider how to deal with the normal interruptions and other occurrences in meditation.

Intrusive thoughts

When thoughts or noises come to mind, observe them, and then label them with titles such as, "thoughts" or "noise." Then choose to return to an awareness of the rise and fall of your abdomen. See the words "in" and "out" with the rise and fall of your abdomen. Sometimes it will be reasonably easy to follow your breath. At other times intrusions will be relentless. When an intrusion is relentless, you can either accept it, or you can try an additional strategy, such as a two-syllable word, as discussed earlier. Repeat it over and over to yourself in your mind, as rapidly as you wish. It will block intrusive thoughts and actually slow down your body's physiology. Two additional calming measures are counting out-breaths and slowing respiration to less than eight breaths per minute.

A second strategy for intrusive thoughts

After you are comfortable with your ability to return to your breath or breath count, then employ this second strategy. Observe your thoughts wherever they go without judging them. When emotions arise, observe those feelings. In this strategy you do not return to concentration on your breath nearly so frequently. You observe your thoughts and strong emotions. In this practice your goal is to follow the path of your thoughts and emotions as an observer.

Strong emotions

If you become disturbed by a feeling, label it and try to stay with the feeling, observing any memories that come to mind until the strong emotion passes. Then choose to turn your attention back to your breathing, noticing the rise and fall of your abdomen, "in," "out," or follow your breath count.

Anger at yourself

It is easy to become annoyed over your inability to stay with your breath even though you know that you are not even supposed to be able to stay with it. We tend to forget that the idea in meditation is not to perfect a blank mind but rather to change our relationship to our thoughts and feelings from an urgent to a peaceful observing stance, the same stance we worked to accomplish in psychoanalysis and psychotherapy. Each time you turn your observing instrument to the rise and fall of your abdomen, something else intrudes. The fact of the matter is that no one can stay with his or her breath. And that is not the point of meditation. The point of meditation is to become comfortable observing, but not acting on, our thoughts and feelings. The key is to be kind and gentle and avoid criticizing yourself over not being able to do the impossible. If you learn this lesson and this lesson alone, meditation will be worthwhile.

Bodily sensations

For many meditators a pain in the body is a very useful focus. Simply let your mind go as you focus on the pain. Later when we learn how to deal with somatic complaints we will use this technique more extensively. Meanwhile, in these moments you may recapture painful and important memories from childhood. Let yourself feel the strong feelings associated with the childhood memory. When the storm passes, let the feelings go.

Sometimes you will be unable to get in touch with anything but the bodily pain or the ache. When that happens, imagine yourself breathing warmth into the area of pain and breathing out the ache or pain. Then let an image of the pain come into your mind. Talk to that image. Ask it what it is trying to tell you. Ask it what you can do for it.

A friend of mine had gout in his left great toe. He thought about the toe and an image of a spinning top came to his mind. He asked the top what it was trying to tell him, and he imagined that the top answered, "You have to do something to keep a top spinning." He asked, "What am I doing?" The top said, "You are putting something in your body every day that keeps me here." He read up on the medicines he was taking and found one that was associated with gout. He called his doctor, who told him to stop the medication. Now he is gout free.

Not all bodily sensations are pain. Itches, tingles, and other sensations come to mind. You may focus upon each of them; then, when the sensation passes, return to your breath.

The impulse to act

There is no better way to remember something that you forgot to do than to begin meditation. Often you will feel a strong impulse to act: make a telephone call, get a cup of coffee, feed the dogs, fix a door handle. You name it, you will feel an urge to do it during meditation.

One action that tempts me repeatedly is the urge to scratch my nose. What I have learned to do is to label this as an "urgency to act." I stay quiet and pay attention to any feelings and memories associated with this impulse. Then if the urge to scratch my nose continues, I slowly, and with concentration on the act, that is, mindfully, scratch my nose.

Notice these two exceptions to following your breath: (1) *Any time strong emotions or memories associated with strong emotions emerge, stay with those feelings until they pass.* (2) *Any time you experience a sensation in your body, focus on that sensation and be aware of the memories that come to mind.* Follow the memories and emotions evoked before you return to your breath. Remember what we are attempting to achieve here. We are attempting to change our relationship to our thoughts and feelings from one in which we experience impulses and feeling as times of urgency to act to times of gentle observation. I cannot remember who said that the hallmark of an educated person is that he can listen to or read anything without becoming frightened or depressed. That is what we are attempting to do in each moment, to become educated to who we really are. Each moment of awareness is a golden moment for rekindling our observing powers. These are the moments that bring us new life after psychotherapy.

Noises

Our next door neighbor, Molly Maher, seems to know when I begin meditation because she sometimes begins chanting. Outsiders might label this barking because Molly is a Wheaton Terrier. I notice this, label it "chanting," and return to my breath.

Intruders

We have a rule in our house that anyone can come into the meditation room at any time and meditate. It is open to all, at any time, night or day. Therefore, intruders happen. Renée, my wife, may come through to tell me about some activity of the day, or Sam and Sarah (our two white poodles) may come in to sit on my lap. Enjoy the interruptions. Then return to meditation.

Times when sitting is not relaxing

Sometimes you may find it expedient to meditate on an exercise machine or on a walk. Sometimes you will find sitting meditation not relaxing. At those times think of the lesson during a repetitive activity such as preparing breakfast or doing the dishes. If you choose to use active times for meditation, the keys are: move deliberately, be aware of your movements, and perform the movements with ceremony and grace. Notice thoughts as they come into your mind. Label them thoughts and focus back on your activity. This way any activity can become meditation practice.

Adding the lesson to breath awareness

When we meditate with a lesson for the day we say the lesson in our mind over the first few breath cycles and the last few. "As for the future, I trust the force."

Ending the meditation

Use a timer. When the timer goes off at the end of your allotted time for meditation, focus on the lesson one more time through several breath cycles. Then, slowly and gently, alert yourself to your surroundings.

Knowing when you are meditating the right way

Any way you meditate is the right way. There is no perfect meditation, nor is there a wrong meditation. When you spend five to forty-five minutes sitting, either following your breath or observing your thoughts and feelings, it is right. The only rule is that you be kind to yourself during the process.

Knowing you are meditating for the right length of time

If the time you choose to meditate feels like it is too long, it is too long. In that circumstance reduce the time that you meditate until you find a time that seems to pass quickly. That is the right length of time.

Experiencing insights in meditation

Although you attempt to calm your mind during meditation to get below the surface noise of your everyday to-do list, there is always something going on in your mind worth noticing. In between returning to your breath or while just following your thoughts, insights will happen, just as they did when you were in psychotherapy. They will happen as you attempt to follow your breath or after meditation, sometimes seemingly out of the blue. They will occur spontaneously. Sometimes they will come frequently, sometimes not; sometimes they come hours after meditation. But they will come, if you give yourself a regular time to practice.

ADVANCED PRACTICE OF INSIGHT MEDITATION

After you have been comfortable following your breath, here is a technique that you can use to enhance your insight about your motivations:

1. Set the timer for twenty minutes.
2. Close your eyes and follow your breath.
3. Each time you have a thought regarding planned action, that is, a thought about something to do right now, think about what came before that thought.

Notice that thoughts of planned action are different from action thoughts. Action thoughts might include all kinds of fantasies. Thoughts of planned action are specifically thoughts that you would act upon if you were not sitting and meditating. See if you can understand how the action thought is linked to the thought that came before it. Then, in addition to that connection, ask yourself about the two component motivations of every thought of planned action, that is, the joining component of the action and the separation component of the action.

I was meditating the other day when I had the thought to telephone one of my patients whom I had started on a new medication. I knew that he would appreciate my concern and I wanted to strengthen our therapeutic bond. That was the joining motivation. I also knew that this particular patient had a tendency to develop unusual side effects to medications and I wanted to head off his complaints at our next visit. That was the separation motive. I wanted to make a preemptive strike to save myself feeling one down during his next visit. Most action thoughts have both motivations, a loving or joining motivation and a competitive or separation motivation.

During the time you meditate you will at times be tempted to look at the clock to see how much time is left. That is a thought about planned action. Each time that happens ask yourself what comes just before that idea to see what thoughts are stimulating the desire to move in you. This attention will allow you to know a lot about what motivates you. Do the same thing with the impulse to shift position or scratch your nose. Each time you have a thought about an action to take right now is a special opportunity to learn about the ideas that move you.

Next let us turn to dealing with symptoms. Remember, at the beginning of the book I described five people who experienced symptoms some time after interrupting their psychotherapy. Phil experienced depression, Janis had symptoms of anger, anxiety, and panic attacks, Bob had obsessive-compulsive symptoms, Father John had somatic symptoms, and Belinda had a return of her disordered habits. There are more possible symptoms, but these cover the majority that might return even after effective psychotherapy.

Part III: Strategies for Healing Symptoms

The symptoms we will address in this part of the book are the ones that we talked about earlier: depression, anxiety, somatization disorders, and habit disorders. Remember that in real life these do not segment themselves so easily. Let's recap our story about John and Greg.

When John returned to find his office moved, he became furious. But he suppressed those feelings because he knew that Greg had intended to reward and not punish him. As the weeks passed he felt more and more isolated from Greg. They no longer met the way they once had at the water cooler. They no longer got each other coffee. They no longer met in the hall so frequently. But John did not let himself feel disappointed for long. Each time he did those angry feelings were replaced by a little nervousness.

John slept poorly. He became worried by his pension plan's erratic performance. He barked at the children and at his wife. He became afraid of flying. He lost his appetite, weight, and an important account. He wondered if he had cancer. His neck hurt. Maybe his cancer had metastasized to the spine. He hated himself for worrying so much. He hated himself for being inattentive to Greg and to his family. He felt fatigued. He drank every day and smoked his pipe even when he did not enjoy it. He thought about suicide. He was depressed.

When angry feelings are suppressed and repressed each time they threaten to surface into consciousness, a small amount of anxiety erupts and repression again pushes the anger out of awareness. We worry about illness. We feel depleted. We are unaware of our option to face our angry feelings and to be at peace with them.

Had John been giving himself the time for introspection or had he been in psychotherapy he might have remembered his experience when his little sister was born. At that time he had been moved out of the windowless nursery next to his parents' room to a room with a view. He was not pleased. He moped around the way he had seen his father mope when he was angry at his mother. Finally, he accepted his being replaced by the "newer model" baby. The way he controlled his angry feelings toward his parents and his sister was to accept the fiction that he must have not lived up to his parents' expectations or they would not have replaced him with his sister. That was the best he could do to figure out what had happened to him. It spared his parents the rage that he felt he would be ostracized for and allowed him to channel his aggression into being a better boy in the future.

That is the way things happen in real life. Symptoms are all mixed together. Sometimes we do not even recognize what is happening to us until we feel depressed. That's why we will start with healing depression.

HEALING DEPRESSION

When we speak of healing here, we mean finding a way to experience peace of mind. In depression you are troubled with anger, but unbeknownst to you that anger turns inward and you hate yourself and you are irritable with others. Think of the spectrum of aggressive emotions as anger, fury, rage, and murderous rage. The turned-inward forms of aggression are guilt, shame, and self-loathing. Here are the two take-home points: (1) *No matter how much you seem to be angry or disappointed with yourself, that blame is really meant for someone else.* (2) *The depressed stance that you adopt in adult life was copied from someone else in your childhood.*

The goal for healing depression is to reverse the process by which you became depressed. First, you recognize your anger at yourself. Then you aim the anger outward toward whom it was originally intended in your adult life. Without acting on the anger you permit yourself to feel the full brunt of your fury toward the person in your adult life for whom the anger was intended. Second, when the anger subsides, you let go of it. You make no attempt to hold on to the angry feelings. Third, when the anger has passed, you ask for the power to let go of any residual resentment. This is forgiveness, and as it is used here, forgiveness means neither condoning nor reconciliation. You might feel just as strong an opposition if the offensive action were repeated. It means merely being willing to drop the burden of resentment that is more a drain on the resenter than the resented. Fourth, you attempt to discover whom that anger was aimed at in your childhood. The theory here is that no intense emotions originate in adult life. Any intense emotion is a holdover from some childhood experience. Then you permit yourself to feel anger at those people in your childhood who hurt you, again without acting on the anger. When the anger subsides you forgive those people. Fifth, you might inquire in your meditation where in your childhood you learned to deal with your anger by being depressed. (Usually becoming depressed is copying someone you observed in childhood.) Then you permit yourself to feel anger at that person for being a poor role model. When the anger subsides you forgive that person.

If all goes well the energy that was expended keeping the anger out of mind and the energy expended being angry are then available for observation. One more area for observation might be fruitful. If all emotions are either love or fear then anger is always a reaction to fear. What is it about the insult that stimulated the depression that is so frightening? It must have been so frightening that you could not let yourself think about it. Now that there is more energy to face your fear think back and find that initial fear. When your fearfulness fades, drop it and get on with life.

In the case of John in our example, he first recognized that he was blaming himself for being thoughtless. Then he discovered that it was really Greg whom he wished to blame for being thoughtless, so he blamed Greg in his mind. He let himself feel furious at Greg for being such a jerk as not to realize that his office's close proximity to

STRATEGIES FOR HEALING SYMPTOMS 37

Greg's was far more important to John than any big, windowed office. He also felt angry at Greg for moving his office without consulting him first. In meditation John attempted to stay with his angry feelings and imagined telling Greg off or even throwing him out of his office window. But, since it is impossible to hold on to any emotion, the more John tried to hold on to his anger the more fleeting it was. The feelings of anger toward Greg faded. When he could no longer feel the bodily sensations of anger, John asked his inner guide to help him let go of the burden of residual resentment toward Greg because it was a burden that was more painful to John than to anyone else. With time the resentment passed. Then, realizing that his reaction to Greg was a major distraction and all major distractions in adult life are recapitulations of childhood traumas, John inquired in his meditation as to who in his childhood had offended him in the way Greg did. His parents came to mind as he remembered when they changed his room after his little sister was born. He let himself feel anger at his parents. When the feelings of anger faded he forgave them. Later he asked himself who in his childhood taught him to be depressed. He remembered his father's moping. He felt angry at his father for teaching him to mope. When his anger faded, he forgave his father. Finally, feeling energetic now, John inquired in his meditation why Greg's actions frightened him so much and he discovered that he was afraid that Greg's moving his office meant that his relationship with Greg would never be the same, the way it had been permanently changed with his parents after his little sister was born. He thought that no matter how hard he worked to be better he would never regain Greg's affection. John realized that he was no longer a child and that he was able to choose to continue a close, cordial relationship with Greg if he wished. He also realized that Greg had no intention of demoting him—quite the opposite. How was Greg to know what had happened in John's childhood? John broke the cycle of depression and of blame.

Daily Practice for Depression

To heal depression, set aside twenty minutes to practice one of the steps in this routine each morning. It is best to meditate in the morning if you can because it will free your energy for the rest of the day. If you cannot meditate in the morning, then meditate whenever you can. Open a journal for writing about the insights you get either during meditation or during the day.

In order to do the exercises that will unburden you from unwanted depressed feelings you should sit comfortably upright in a chair and either close your eyes or keep them slightly open and unfocused but aimed at a place on the floor about six to eight feet in front of you. Plant both feet firmly on the floor. Feel solid and anchored. Put your hands on your legs. Breathe regularly from the diaphragm so that when you inhale your abdomen expands and when you exhale your abdomen contracts. Imagine "In" on the in-breath and "Out" on the out-breath. Pay attention only to your breath, that is, only to the rise and fall of your abdomen. Notice that when you pay attention only to your breath you feel at peace. Some people cannot breathe while moving their abdomen, that is, they cannot let their abdomen expand with an in-breath and contract with an out-breath. If you are one of these people then just notice your breath at your nostrils. Repeat this in your mind over several breath cycles: *With this in-breath I relax my body, with this out-breath I relax my mind.*

Depression is my teacher.

First remember that depression is good because it allows you to slow down and reexamine your priorities. It gives you a chance to look into yourself and see how your mind works. So do not keep the cycle of hate going by hating your depression. Embrace your depression as an old friend who has something to teach you. Remember that this emotion is your unconscious mind telling you that this is the time for you to put yourself in neutral, to examine the direction your choices are taking you, to either renew your determination or to change direction. Use your depression as an opportunity to slow down and give yourself some time to think. *Depression is my teacher.* Write this on a card that you carry around during the day. Several times during the day look at the card and be at peace. Now begin your daily meditation with this lesson.

At the end of the day write on your card or in your journal any ideas that come to mind about what you can learn from your depression.

Depression is anger turned on myself.

Depression is based on your looking at something that happened in the past and hating yourself for what you did. In the case of John, he thinks of his thoughtless behavior toward his wife and children. He thinks of his anger at Greg and blames himself for being thoughtless. This blame is based on his childhood story. In his childhood story he is to blame for the rejection that he experienced when his sister was born. In his meditation he asks himself who is it he would blame for being thoughtless if he were not blaming himself.

This meditation exercise has two parts. In part one you let yourself be angry at yourself. In part two you redirect that anger outside yourself.

1. After several breath cycles ask yourself to discover what you are blaming yourself for. Let yourself be angry with yourself. Put the blame in as clear a picture as you can. Stay with that feeling of anger toward yourself until the physical sensations of the emotion fade.
2. When the feelings of self blame subside ask yourself, "If I am not really angry at myself, who is this anger really meant for?" Usually a person in your daily life pops to mind. Then let yourself feel the full strength of your angry feelings toward that person. Stay with these feelings as long as you can. Imagine telling this person how you dislike him, how he has let you down. When you do this, you will see that eventually the physical sensations associated with the emotion of anger fade. When they fade, return to your breath and feel peace. At the end of meditation say to yourself over several breath cycles, *With this in-breath I relax my body, with this out-breath I relax my mind.* Stay with that thought for a minute or so.

After meditation write this lesson on a card. Several times during the day, hourly if that is convenient, look at the lesson: *Depression is anger turned on myself.* Spend a minute following your breath.

At the end of the day write on your card or in your journal any further insights you have regarding the day's lesson.

Angry feelings begin my healing journey.

Far from being a bad thing, angry feelings and fantasies are good because they begin the healing process. If we accept our angry feelings as a normal, healthy part of ourselves we will be taking the first step on the road to peace of mind. Today begin practice with the same routine as yesterday. Begin by saying to yourself, *With this in-breath I relax my body, with this out-breath I relax my mind.* After you are relaxed for several breath cycles recall your angry feelings aimed at the person other than yourself from the day before. Let yourself feel the anger again, not at yourself but at the other person. See if the angry feelings are as strong as they were the day before. If they are, stay with them until their physical sensations fade. When they do say to yourself: *Angry feelings begin my healing journey.* Spend a minute following your breath.

After meditation write this lesson on a card. Several times during the day, hourly if that is convenient, look at the lesson: *Angry feelings begin my healing journey.* Spend a minute following your breath.

At the end of the day write any additional insights you have regarding angry feelings on your card or in your journal.

Forgiveness paves the road to peace of mind.

Today, the fourth day of depression practice, begin with the same routine. Begin by saying to yourself, *With this in-*

breath I relax my body, with this out-breath I relax my mind. After you are relaxed for several breath cycles let yourself get in touch with any feelings of guilt, embarrassment, or self-loathing. Feel the feelings strongly. Then ask for whom is this anger really meant. Another person in your daily life or someone from your past may pop into mind. Allow yourself to feel angry at that person with every ounce of energy you can muster. Stay with the feeling.

When the physical sensations associated with the emotion fade, ask for the power to release your feelings of frustration and disappointment. Ask for the power to forgive. Asking for the power is like a prayer. Prayer, in this sense, does not mean one has to believe in God. In fact, prayer works whether you believe in God or not. If you believe in God you may choose to pray to God, or to the Holy Spirit, or to a Higher Power. You may choose to pray to the ultimate force in the universe or to your own reasoned intuition. It doesn't matter. Prayer works. Trust yourself. Say, *Forgiveness paves the road to peace of mind* over several breath cycles.

With time, frustration will fade and peace will take its place. Do not expect that resentment will disappear immediately, but if you are willing to accept the help of the force within you, your inner guide, it will disappear. This is forgiveness. Forgiveness does not mean condoning. In fact, you may oppose them if that person were to repeat the actions that stirred up your hurt and hate. Forgiveness also does not mean reconciliation. You may or may not choose to make up with the person you forgive. Forgiveness means being willing to let go of the burden of resentment, which is always more a burden for the hater than for the hated. It is the hater who has the burden. Forgiveness relieves that burden. At the end of your practice session say for several breath cycles again, *Forgiveness paves the road to peace of mind.* When you have finished meditation, write the lesson for the day on a card that you can carry with you throughout the day. Every hour or so calm yourself and follow your breath for one minute. Repeat the lesson at the end of the minute: *Forgiveness paves the road to peace of mind.*

At the end of the day write any additional insights you have regarding forgiveness on your card or in your journal.

I am never angry at the person I think.

On the fifth day begin practice with the same routine. Begin by saying to yourself, *With this in-breath I relax my body, with this out-breath I relax my mind.* After you are relaxed for several breath cycles, say the following through several more breath cycles: *I am never angry at the person I think.* Ask to become aware of the person or persons in your past whom the persons in your life today remind you of. Here you are invoking the theory that all strong emotions come from childhood and that anyone you feel really irritated by in adult life is a stand-in for an influential person in your childhood whom you have not forgiven. Ask for that person to come to mind. A picture of your mother, father, sister, brother, grandmother, grandfather, uncle, or aunt may come to mind. Again, let yourself feel all the frustration at that person that you can muster. Imagine telling that person how you feel. When your enthusiasm for anger wanes, ask for the power to forgive that person. Do this even if you do not feel that the person deserves forgiveness, because forgiveness is not for that person, it is for you. If you harbor hate, you are the one who is burdened, and you are praying for relief from that burden. At the end of your practice say over several breath cycles, *I am never angry at the person I think.*

When you have finished meditation, write the lesson for the day on a card that you can carry with you throughout the day. Every hour or so calm yourself and follow your breath for one minute. Repeat the lesson at the end of the minute: *I am never angry at the person I think.*

At the end of the day write any additional insights you have regarding forgiveness on your card or in your journal.

Whoever suffers is not me.

On the sixth day practice the same routine. Begin by saying to yourself, *With this in-breath I relax my body, with this out-breath I relax my mind.* After you are relaxed for several breath cycles, say the following through several more breath cycles: *Whoever suffers is not me.*

Most of us learn to be depressed by copying the example of someone in our childhood. When we were children we could not complain about the caregiver's depressive behavior for fear of losing the nurturing from that person, so we learned to copy the depressed behavior. Let the person come to mind who taught you to be depressed. When that person comes to mind, blame him or her for being a faulty role model. Then when the feeling of blame fades, ask for the power to forgive that person. At the end of your practice say over several breath cycles, *Whoever suffers is not me.* When you have finished meditation, write the lesson for the day on a card that you can carry with you throughout the day. Every hour or so calm yourself and follow your breath for one minute. Repeat the lesson at the end of the minute: *Whoever suffers is not me.*

At the end of the day write any additional insights you have regarding forgiveness on your card or in your journal.

All emotions are either love or fear.

Repeat in your mind over several breath cycles: *With this in-breath I relax my body, with this out-breath I relax my mind.* After you are relaxed for several breath cycles, say the following through several more breath cycles: *All emotions are either love or fear.* Then think back to the incidents that stimulated your depression in adult life. Think of the person or persons who hurt you. Think of what they did and one at a time ask yourself, "Why did this frighten me?" After meditation use a journal to write down in as much detail as you can how their actions frightened you. Make a special effort to write what personality characteristics the person who frustrated you displayed. For example, "When Greg moved my office without asking me he seemed to be treating me just like my parents did when my little sister was born. They showed absolutely no hint of recognition that I would experience the distance of our rooms as abandonment. I remember having nightmares, probably so I could crawl in bed with them, but would my father let me—oh no. What a self-centered, uncaring jerk he was. I was afraid that Greg's actions started a cold war like I felt I had with my father from the day he and my mother moved my room. But I am an adult now and I can choose to remain close to Greg even though he misunderstands me. I do not have to be ruled by my fear as I was in childhood." After you have written your fears in as much detail as possible return to a relaxed state by saying to yourself: *All emotions are either love or fear.* After several breath cycles feel at peace.

Write the lesson for the day on a card that you can carry with you throughout the day. Every hour or so calm yourself and follow your breath for one minute. Repeat the lesson at the end of the minute: *All emotions are either love or fear.*

At the end of the day write any additional insights you have regarding forgiveness on your card or in your journal.

Oneness is the optimal view.

In the final analysis what is really to blame in all psychological symptoms whether we suffer depression, anxiety, bodily symptoms, or habit disorders is the limited capability of our own perceptual system. Our perceptions tell us that we are all separate from one another but that is not true. Greg's actions were frightening and stimulated anger because John experienced him as separate and threatening. John did not recognize Greg as a part of him, someone with whom he was as connected as we are with each person in a dream of ours. That person is not an independent entity but a stand-in for part of our childhood story, that is, a character in the story that we invented to explain our feelings when we were little and did not have the ability to understand adult motives and limitations. In a very real sense Greg is John's teacher because he gave John an opportunity to look into himself and to see how his childhood experience was distorting his adult experience.

Our senses play tricks on us. They tell us that we are separate but that is not so. Physicists tell us that we are exchanging millions of atoms with each other each time we breathe out and in. So we are all connected. If we could see ourselves at a distance and over longer periods of time we could see how our interactions affect everyone we come in contact with. And then our kindness or our irritability spreads. So we have a choice to teach kindness and compassion or irritability. It is our choice and it affects every person we come in contact with every day.

Any time we choose compassion over conflict we heal ourselves. If someone is irritable with you today extend yourself in kindness and compassion and see how much better you feel for it. You will heal the other person and heal yourself.

At the end of meditation today write on a card: *Oneness is the optimal view*. Write the lesson for the day on a card that you can carry with you throughout the day. Every hour or so calm yourself and follow your breath for one minute. Repeat the lesson at the end of the minute: *Oneness is the optimal view*.

At the end of the day write on your card or in your journal any additional insights you have regarding forgiveness.

If you are not currently in psychotherapy, and if after going through these exercises once you do not feel better, try them again. If you still feel very depressed call your therapist for some additional help.

HEALING ANXIETY

Remember our story about John and Greg? Well let's suppose it went a bit differently. John entered his office after a vacation to find that he had been moved from the office adjoining his boss, Greg, to a big office with windows down the hall. He was immediately furious. He knew that it would not be politic to go ranting down the hallway, cursing the gods, so he pushed down his angry feelings. He became anxious that he might spout off in some way that would further alienate him from his boss, so he put a smile on his face and calmly knocked on Greg's door. His boss and mentor answered the door, smiling broadly.

"Surprise! How does it feel to finally have a decent-sized office with windows?" Greg asked.

John knew now that he was not being punished but rewarded. How could he have been so angry with Greg?

"Great, just great! Thank you very much."

As the weeks passed John felt more and more isolated from Greg. They no longer met at the water cooler. They no longer got each other coffee. They no longer shared sidewalk consultations as frequently as they had before. John was angry at Greg but he did not let himself feel those feelings for long. Each time he did, he felt a little nervous, then the angry feelings went away.

John thought he was fine, but he began to worry about finances and his children's safety. He thought Jane was spending too much money. He also worried about the children's being kidnapped on the way home from school. He insisted that Jane take elaborate security precautions so nothing bad would happen to the little ones. One night John developed chest pain. He began gasping for breath. Jane called 911 and he was taken to the hospital. All his tests were normal. John had had a panic attack. He was a nervous wreck and he had no idea why.

John had developed an anxiety disorder with symptoms of generalized anxiety and panic attacks. He did not let himself get angry at Greg, but his annoyance came out at his wife, disguised as worries about finances and worries about her child care. If he were in psychotherapy he might have been helped to recognize that he was angry at Greg and that this anger harkened back to his anger at his parents for moving him away from their room when his baby sister was born. He feared that if he showed his anger to his parents he would further alienate them. He was convinced that he must have been bad in the first place or they would not have acquired a new baby. He would have remembered his fear of going to school and his worries that some robber would enter the house and steal his baby sister away. He would have discovered that his worries as a child were a cover for his aggressive wishes that someone would harm his parents and his little sister for what they had done to him.

Anxiety is a feeling of impending calamity. Sigmund Freud said that all feelings of calamity in adult life parallel those of childhood where there are four basic fears: loss of the object,[1] loss of the object's love, castration,[2] and loss of the approval from one's own conscience. So when we feel anxiety, if we look deeply into ourselves we will experience one or a combination of these fears.

Freud also said that each fear disguises a wish for retaliation. Fear of loss of the object disguises a retaliatory wish to kill the object. Fear of loss of the object's love partially disguises a retaliatory wish to reject the object. Fear of castration partially disguises the retaliatory wish to cas-

---

1. The object is the loved one whom the child depends on for the sustenance that is necessary for life itself.
2. Castration means retaliation from the object's jealous mate who does not like the object paying so much attention to the child.

trate one's rival, and fear of loss of the approval of one's conscience partially disguises the wish to rebel against the conscience.

Let's examine each one in more detail. Do you remember the first time you had a crush on someone who did not return your affection? Do you remember the misery it caused you? This is similar to loss of the object. I had a friend, Gary, who was in love with Sally Pittman, a girl in our sixth grade class. One Sunday Gary asked me to go with him to the Anderson Public Library, knowing that Sally would be there. He sought her out. But Sally was not interested in talking to him. She was talking to another boy a grade ahead of us. She made it clear she was not interested in Gary. Gary could not talk to me. He was crushed. He tried to hide the tears in his eyes. He thought that Sally was the only girl for him and that no one else could make him feel safe and whole. Those feelings are similar to an infant's dependency on his mother. He knew that Sally was lost to him. In his devastation, Gary sat down and wrote a term paper on myocardial infarction, a suitable topic for a boy with a broken heart.

We would all like to avoid that crushed feeling. If we feel threatened that we may be on the verge of experiencing it, we may feel intense anxiety, which works in part to disguise our feelings of anger at the lost object. In Gary's case he turned to action—writing—which helped him use his aggressive energy on a subject related to his experience—heart attacks—and it helped him ward off his feared loss of ability to function as a person.

Loss of the object's love is similar to the feeling of loss of the object, but loss of the object has a finality to it, whereas loss of the object's love holds some hope for reinstatement of a formerly held position of affection. Remember breaking up with a girlfriend or boyfriend in early adolescence and how miserable you felt until you had reestablished the relationship by making up? The period of time when you feared that you had lost the love of the other is what it feels like to experience fear of loss of the object's love. It is intense misery, but there is hope; because you had an established relationship at some time, there is hope of reinstatement. Fear of loss of the object's love can also trigger feelings of jealousy. Some people, however, are so afraid of feeling a loss of love that they are unable to feel jealousy. If we are unable to feel jealousy then we will be unable to know or understand how we evoke jealousy in others. To be unable to feel jealousy can be a crippling lack that can make a mess of relationships as easily as can feeling jealous over every little thing. Rather than having jealous feelings, a person may deny them and busy himself doing something like Gary did when he wrote his term paper on myocardial infarction. Instead of feeling jealousy, a person may feel a generalized feeling of dread, not knowing where it comes from, or may feel panic associated with something that has only a symbolic connection to the fear. A person may become afraid of spiders, or heights, or going out of the house, not realizing that what he fears out of the house is seeing the object of his jealousy walking in the mall with someone else.

    Fear of castration, or its analog, fear of emotional impotence, means a fear of someone else lopping off your ability to be a competitive force in your life. A colleague of mine, David, worked on a research project at the National Institutes of Mental Health. He was attempting to prevent suicidal gestures in military enlisted men during the Vietnam War. Suicidal gestures were very frequent in men who feared being sent to Vietnam and once a person made a suicidal gesture he was very likely to do it over and over again because the gesture was usually by overdose of some drug like diazepam that left the person without any memory of his overdose when it wore off. David's research team developed a pioneering means of addressing the problem by setting up videotaping equipment in the emergency room that helped remind the person who overdosed of the misery that led to the suicidal behavior. Once the person remembered, then the feelings could be dealt with in psychotherapy. The rate of recurrence dropped dramatically.

Fear of the disapproval of our own conscience is perhaps the most insidious cause of anxiety. We can fear punishment from our conscience if we *do* something wrong, but even more disturbing is when we feel danger of being punished by our conscience if we even *think* something aggressive or if we *aspire* to some grand ideal. Even more disturbing than that, we may be punished by our conscience if we do something well. I had a suitemate in college who was a terrific student. Jim did exceptionally well, especially on complex examinations because those were opportunities for him to use his extraordinary synthetic abilities. That is, he could pull together vast amounts of information in ways that normal people just could not match. Yet, after each examination, when he broke the curve, he would be miserable. He felt so down he would get drunk to try to ward off his misery. Then he felt remorse over getting drunk. I do not know what was behind his fear of showing his extraordinary ability, but I know that his conscience was giving him a terrible time. To escape the terror of his conscience for using his gift, he got drunk.

When we suffer from anxiety, one or a combination of these fears is in play. But, there is one more important factor: just as depression is about something we have done in the past, anxiety is about something we fear in the future. Therefore, any time we are in the present we will not feel anxiety if we follow our breath. There is one exception to this rule and that is when something sets off our physiology so that it seems to be operating independently from our mind. A good way to tell when that is happening is when our heart is racing and it does not slow down when we relax our body and mind. A friend, Mike, was undergoing cardiac rehabilitation after bypass surgery. He told me that he had a run of atrial tachycardia while he was hooked up to a cardiac monitor. It took him a long time to stop his heart from racing by use of his relaxation and meditation techniques. During the period of racing heart beats he imagined that his marriage was over, that his wife did not love him any more, that his business would be in chapter 11 within six months, that he was making terrible business decisions, and that it did not much matter because even if all went well, he would die soon. When the atrial tachycardia stopped he felt completely at peace. He loved his wife and she loved him, his business was in a normal cycle, he had done all the right things to protect it, and he was looking forward to a nice Thanksgiving with his daughter and his grandchildren. Although it is possible that his run of atrial tachycardia could have been stimulated by anxiety, in this case it seemed that a physiological irritant started the process and physiological change, possibly induced by meditation, stopped the heart racing and the anxiety.

The problem with anxiety is that when it is working the way it is intended, we have no clue about what is causing it. We can be sure that often what comes to mind first is probably not it. The reason we can be so sure is that anxiety pushes its cause out of mind. So we have to be less anxious before we can figure out what the anxiety is all about. Therefore step 1 is to become less anxious. Using meditation, we start with the knowledge that if we follow our breath and stay in the present we cannot feel anxious because anxiety is about the future.

Daily Practice for Healing Anxiety

If you are experiencing symptoms of anxiety similar to those outlined above here is a self-help approach.

Each morning before breakfast set aside twenty minutes to practice one of the steps in this routine. It is best to meditate in the morning if you can because it will free your energy for the rest of the day. If you cannot meditate in the morning, then meditate whenever you can.

In order to do the exercises that will unburden you from feelings of anxiety you should sit comfortably upright in a chair and either close your eyes or keep them slightly open and unfocused, but aimed at a place on the floor about six to eight feet in front of you. Plant both feet firmly on the floor. Feel solid and anchored. Put your hands on your legs. Breathe regularly from the diaphragm so that when you inhale your abdomen expands and when you exhale your abdomen contracts. Imagine "In" on the in-breath and "Out" on the out-breath. Pay attention only to your breath, that is only to the rise and fall of your abdomen. Notice that when you pay attention only to your breath you feel at peace. Some people cannot breathe while moving their abdomen, that is, they cannot let their abdomen expand with an in-breath and contract with an out-breath. If you are one of these people then just notice your breath at your nostrils. Repeat this in your mind: *With this in-breath I relax my body, with this out-breath I relax my mind.*

Anxiety begins my healing journey.

The first step is to remember that anxiety is an opportunity to discover something that is threatening to you. Anxiety is a signal that brings repression to work to put out of mind what is really bothering you so you will focus on something that is not a real danger. This is different than fear, which is in response to an actual external danger. Anxiety is your friend because it is a beacon to healing work. It gives you a chance to do something good for yourself.

The first step is calming yourself. I recommend using a mantra when you are really revved up. A good one for me is "trutfo-gaypax." It is nonsense but to me it stands for "when I trust the force, I gain peace." It means that I can turn the problem over to my reasoned intuition and admit that I cannot handle it by my will alone. I need the help of my inspired unconscious mind to help me get past the anxiety. I let the mantra play over and over in my mind at its own pace. That usually lets me find a deeper relaxation than I can without a mantra.

I do not know what distresses me.

Again the first step is calming yourself. Often a mantra is useful to get calm. I use "trutfo-gaypax," which stands for "when I trust the force, I gain peace." When you feel calm, try to get yourself to realize that the worries on your mind are not the basis for your anxiety by saying over several breath cycles, *I do not know what distresses me.*

Then try to follow your breath and to become peaceful by staying in the present. At the very end of meditation ask for help in discovering what hidden grievance lies behind your anxiety. Then use a notebook and write whatever comes to mind for about ten minutes. Then put the notebook away until evening. Write on a card that you will look at several times this day, *I do not know what distresses me*. Each time you look at the card calm yourself and follow your breath for a minute or two.

In the evening meditate again, repeating the same procedure. At the end of meditation look at your notebook. Read what you wrote in the morning and add any additional insights to what you have written. Over a period of time those you are angry at and the reasons why will emerge in your notebook.

My stressors are grievances in my mind.

The next day begin your meditation with a mantra that works for you. When you have calmed your mind and body, say to yourself over several breath cycles: *My stressors are grievances in my mind*. Grievances are the wrongs we imagine others have done to us. One way to get in touch with your grievances is just to follow your breath. In between moving back to the rise and fall of your abdomen your grievances will pop into mind. Or later in the day when you are thinking about something else a grievance will come to mind. Either after meditation in the morning, evening, or both, write any grievances that come to mind.

At the very end of meditation ask for guidance in writing in your notebook. Write whatever comes to mind about grievances. Write your grievances in the notebook because the things that make us angry are the things we fear.

After your meditation and writing write on a card, *My stressors are grievances in my mind.* You know what to do with the card.

Meditate in the evening again. And review your notebook afterwards.

I can feel peace instead of conflict.

On day three of the anxiety healing cycle remind yourself that any time you focus on your breath or your mantra you are at peace. Actually, any time you focus your attention on what is happening at the moment you feel peace whether you are listening intently, or watching intently, or doing something intently. When Gary wrote his paper on myocardial infarction, he was doing something intently to establish peace. So living in the present moment is the key to peace of mind. If you are able to take pleasure in ordinary activities you will be at peace. Practice doing any chore. My favorite is taking spots out of a rug. I get my spray bottle of Resolve and a clean white cloth and turn my attention to any rug in the house or in my office. I do not let anyone else in my office remove spots from the carpeting because no one else wants to do it, and no one enjoys it as much as I do. It is linked in my mind with earlier times when my sons Michael and Jeffrey were little and we were the "Spot Swat Team." When we found a spot on the carpet, it gave us each the opportunity to have a pail of cloths and a spray bottle of cleaner, and, like a well oiled spot-removing machine, we made short the life of that dreaded spot. We made such a game of it that removing spots is something I still enjoy a lot. In meditation I traced that pleasure back to my Grandma Kempf. There were times when we did the same thing at her house but there it was removing spots from the wallpaper. We all had our bucket and cloths and some petroleum-smelling, puttylike material that we rubbed on the spots on the wallpaper. I could help with that chore when I was very young and not much good for other things like washing dishes or vacuuming.

So meditate with this thought at the beginning and end of meditation: *I can feel peace instead of conflict.* At the end of the meditation write this lesson on a card. Take a few minutes to write in your notebook after meditation. Take several times during the day to remind yourself of the power of living in the present.

Meditate in the evening as well. Make additions to your notebook each evening.

Forgiveness paves the road to peace of mind.

Today remind yourself of the power of forgiveness. Remember that forgiveness is mostly for yourself, although it is bound to change your demeanor so that it will help anyone you have contact with as well. Forgiveness just means being willing to give up the burden of resentment. But remember you cannot do this by willpower alone. You need help from the guiding force within you. Also, remember that first you must blame, even if only for an instant, before you can forgive someone, so blame away. Search for any resentment toward anyone in your life, past or present. See if there is some anger toward someone who has disappointed you. Let that resentment build. Then, as you let yourself feel it, it will dissipate because emotions that are not warded off come and go. When the bodily sensation accompanying anger is gone, ask for the power to forgive those people you blamed. That is, ask for the power to let go of the residual resentment left behind from your angry feelings. There is nothing wrong with feeling and thinking blame. It is only trying to push blame out of mind that is a problem because pushing blame out of mind is a surefire way to keep anxiety alive. So open yourself to blaming thoughts and feelings. Anxiety is the signal that mobilizes the forces of the mind to push blame out of mind. Blame is good because it is the first step to peace of mind.

After meditation write on the card you will carry today, *Forgiveness paves the road to peace of mind.*

Meditate in the evening as well. Review your notebook and make any additions to those you wish to blame and forgive in the notebook.

I have projected the world I see.

Many of the injuries we imagine others have done to us are injuries we wish to inflict on others but we are afraid of those wishes, so we suppress them and then we project them onto others. That way we can say, "It is not I who am hostile, it's the other guy." That may be the attraction of action movies. "It is not I who want to blow up my enemies. It's Rambo. I can enjoy the process of blowing up enemies without actually acknowledging my own wishes. I create ogres in my imagination so I do not have to acknowledge my own hostile wishes." In this exercise go ahead and be Rambo in your imagination. Ambush the people you wish to get even with in your imagination. Then, when your angry feelings dissipate, let them go and return to peace.

After meditation write on a card: *I have projected the world I see.* Look at that card several times each day and each time you do be still for an instant. Follow your breath and return to peace. Look at your notebook and write what comes to mind.

Oneness is the optimal view.

Most of our anxiety arises because we feel separate from the people and world around us. If we could see our connectedness in each moment of our life we would know that we have nothing to fear but our own projected hostility. Each moment of the day we are using the tools others have made for us to make our lives easier. From the keyboard I am typing on right this second to the light bulb that illuminates it, to the screen on my computer, to the central processing unit, to the WordPerfect® software—all these components were made by people, thousands and thousands of them, and I am connected to them through the products of their work and talent. We do not have to be able to experience a connection at a subatomic level where we know we are sharing atoms with each living creature on this planet. All we have to do is stop and think. Think about the clothes we are wearing, the air we are breathing, the food we eat, the beverage we drink. All are brought to us by others, connected to us through their efforts, here with us in the history of the articles around us, right now, helping us in innumerable ways.

We can be facilitators of productivity any time we choose compassion over conflict. If someone is irritable with you today see that person as frightened and calling out for help. Extend yourself in the brotherhood of man. Extend yourself with understanding rather than copying the other person's irritability. You will feel peaceful yourself and you will bring peace to the other person. You will facilitate the productivity of the other person and facilitate your own productivity as well.

At the end of meditation today write on a card: *Oneness is the optimal view.*

Meditate in the evening as well. Review your notebook in the morning and evening.

At the end of these exercises, if your anxiety is under control move on. If not repeat the cycle again.

HEALING PAIN AND WORRIES ABOUT MY BODY

Pain and worries about your body are often a sign that you harbor some angry feelings that are unacceptable to you. Rather than feeling the anger you repress it and feel muscle and joint pains, back pains, headaches, indigestion, heartburn, or irritable bowel symptoms instead of anger.

A woman with two young children gave up practicing medicine to raise her children because in her family childrearing took precedence over everything else. She developed back pain. When I suggested to her that she may have feelings outside her awareness about her recent decision to give up her medical practice, she denied it and sought medical treatment for her back. A year later after exhaustive medical treatment she was in more pain and was scheduled for back surgery for an extruded lumbar disk. She returned to me to try again to find other components to her pain. Only then did she begin to recognize her angry feelings toward her husband, her children, and her parents, all of whom she experienced as expecting her to give up her profession. As she became aware of her angry feelings her back pain subsided without surgery.[3]

To make an inventory about your fears that may contribute to physical symptoms, get a notebook and make notes each day after meditation.

Painful bodily sensations and worry about your body are often disguised feelings of anxiety and anger but these emotions are coded as aches, pains, and other bodily sensations. Always get a thorough examination from your physician to rule out organic disease before working on healing yourself. Abide by his recommendations. Do not turn your back on medical science. Do not throw down your crutches and walk without them if you have a broken leg. Use this section to attend to the emotional dimension of any physical illness. Or if no physical illness can be identified then use this section to attend to your aches, pains, repressed anger, and worries about your body.

I will search my body as a window to my mind.

The tool most useful to begin meditation is the body inventory. In this process you search each part of your body for tension and pain. Here is the way it works.

1. In a sitting or lying position begin attending to your breath. Most people find lying down an optimal position for doing a body inventory.
2. Imagine your breath flowing in your nose and through your body to your left toes, foot, ankle, calf,

---

3. A thorough treatment of the discoveries made regarding back pain and its treatment may be found in Dr. John E. Sarno's book *Healing Back Pain*, New York: Warner Books, 1991.

knee, thigh, and pelvis. Focus on each area from thirty seconds to one minute. As you breathe in, picture sparkling oxygen molecules as bright little "Os" zipping through your body to the area of bodily attention. As you breathe out, imagine sparkling molecules of carbon dioxide flowing out into the atmosphere where plants may use them as a source of energy.
3. Move to your right toes, foot, ankle, calf, knee, thigh, and pelvis.
4. Move to your lower back, abdomen, chest, upper back, and neck.
5. Move to your left fingers, forearm, elbow, arm, and shoulder.
6. Focus on your right fingers, forearm, elbow, arm, and shoulder. From your neck move over the top of your head to your face and back down to the center of your chest. End your search by allowing a bright white light to fill your chest with feelings of love and kindness. Let the warmth begin in the middle of your body at the junction of your abdomen and chest. Then let the white, warm light of love spread to your chest, then abdomen, then limbs, until you imagine your whole body aglow with loving kindness.
7. If at any time in your body search you feel pain or discomfort or a strong emotion associated with a bodily sensation, let your attention stay in that area for a while. Open yourself to the experience of pain or discomfort rather than trying to avoid it. Face the feelings, thoughts, and sensations associated with the discomfort. When the memories and emotions fade, move on. If they do not fade, stay

with them to the end of your meditation period. Anxiety is an emotion that stirs us to move away. If we do not move away but face the emotions and sensations and memories behind the anxiety, anxiety will fade as will any bodily sensations that are anxiety-produced.

Another technique is to let the bodily discomfort form an image in your mind like the image of the spinning top of the man with gout. Ask that image what the pain is trying to tell you. Ask the image what you can do for it.

At the end of meditation write this on a card that you look at several times each day: *I will search my body as a window to my mind*. Each time you look at the card be still for a moment. Search your body and feel your bodily sensations. Breathe healing "Os" into your pain and breathe out "CO_2s" to nurture the plant life on our planet.

A man who was experiencing irritable bowel symptoms noticed in his body search that when he got to his left knee he felt pain there. A memory emerged of playing catch with his grandfather in the back yard. His grandfather became angry that he was throwing the ball too hard and threw the ball back to him harder than he was able to catch. The ball hit him in the left knee and he doubled over in pain. His grandfather walked away in disgust. He feared the loss of his grandfather's love so he apologized to his grandfather and tried to make up. As he was conducting his body search he realized that he had swallowed all his angry feelings about being hurt by his grandfather. The memory paralleled an experience in his present life where he was attempting to accommodate a supervisor who was inflicting painful restrictions on his productive work behavior. In his meditation he was able to face his angry feeling toward both his grandfather and his supervisor and he was able to recognize his fear that he would be left without support if he did not seek their approval. Acknowledging his feelings gave him the emotional energy to deal with the disruptive work situation. His irritable bowel symptoms subsided. When they return now, he knows that it is time to use the body search to root out his repressed anger and fears.

Think of bodily pain as a signal that your body has some e-mail for you. Then listen to your body talk and decode the message.

After your body inventory turn to your notebook and write any worries about your body that came to mind during your meditation. Write what came to mind when you formed an image of your pain. Write the answer to your question about what your pain was trying to tell you. Write the answer to your question about what you could do for your pain. Repeat this exercise each day until your angry feelings and your worries come to the surface. Once you have identified the emotions coded by your bodily sensations, deal with them by the following exercises.

My stressors are grievances in my mind.

The next day begin your meditation with the following: *With this in-breath I relax my body, with this out-breath I relax my mind.* Say this to yourself over several breath cycles until you feel yourself relax. When you have calmed your mind and body say to yourself over several breath cycles, *My stressors are grievances in my mind.* Grievances are the wrongs we imagine others have done to us. One way to get in touch with your grievances is just to follow your breath. In between moving back to the rise and fall of your abdomen your grievances will pop into mind. If a bodily sensation comes to mind, focus on that and see if any grievance is hidden behind the bodily sensation. Or later in the day when you are thinking about an ache or a pain, a grievance will come to mind. Either after meditation in the morning, evening, or both, write any grievances that come to mind.

At the very end of meditation ask for guidance in writing in your notebook. Write whatever comes to mind about grievances. Write your grievances in your notebook because the things that make you angry are the things you fear.

After your meditation and writing write on a card, *My stressors are grievances in my mind.* You know what to do with the card.

Meditate in the evening again and review your notebook afterward.

Angry feelings begin my healing journey.

Angry feelings are good. Being able to identify your angry feelings and sit with them without acting on them is perhaps the master aptitude for physical and emotional well-being. Nothing predicts the success of attitudinal healing more than your ability to recognize and face your angry feelings. In this meditation ask that any angry feeling buried in your unconscious mind be revealed to you so that you can face those feelings in your peaceful meditation without acting on them and without using the feelings to stimulate planned action. Ask for the strength to sit with your angry feelings until they subside because if you do not attempt to avoid these feelings they will subside and they will no longer stimulate tension in your body.

At the very end of meditation write in your notebook. Write whatever comes to mind about angry feelings.

After your meditation and writing write on a card, *Angry feelings begin my healing journey.* You know what to do with the card.

Meditate in the evening again and review your notebook afterward.

Forgiveness paves the road to peace of mind.

On this day remind yourself of the power of forgiveness. Remember that forgiveness is mostly for yourself although it is bound to change your demeanor so it will help anyone you have contact with as well. Forgiveness just means being willing to give up the burden of resentment. But remember you cannot do this yourself. You need help from the guiding force within you. Also, remember that first you must blame, even if only for an instant, before you can forgive someone, so blame away. Search for any resentment toward anyone in your life past or present. See if there is some anger toward someone who has disappointed you. Let that resentment build. Then as you let yourself feel it, it will dissipate because emotions come and go. When it is gone, ask for the power to forgive those people you blamed. That is, ask for the power to let go of the residual resentment left behind from your angry feelings. There is nothing wrong with feeling and thinking blame. It is only trying to push blame out of mind that is a problem because pushing blame out of mind is a surefire way to keep anxiety around. So open yourself to blaming thoughts and feelings. Anxiety is the signal that mobilizes the forces of the mind to push blame out of mind. Blame is good because it is the first step to peace of mind.

After meditation write on the card you will carry today, *Forgiveness paves the road to peace of mind.*

Meditate in the evening as well. Review your notebook and make any additions in the notebook to those you wish to blame.

Oneness is the optimal view.

Today your healing journey offers you a new opportunity. You may choose to see yourself connected with those around you rather than separate from them. Look at the moon or the sky. Think about all the people who are looking at the moon or sky right now. You are connected with these people through your perceptions. You share your perceptions with those around you. Frequently I hear from my co-workers, "Lake Michigan is really gorgeous today. Did you see the green hues as the clouds drifted by this morning?" "I did and yesterday the water was so blue and so clear that the horizon looked like it was painted on with an eyebrow pencil, just a perfect dark line between the water and the sky." The ever-changing pictures of nature in all its beauty are perceptions we share. They unite us in the community of man. Feel that unity and when the opportunity arises extend yourself in kindness and compassion to someone in your world today. A few friendly words on an elevator, helping someone cross the street or get out of a car, or offering directions to someone who seems lost. All these moments are opportunities to celebrate the connectedness of perceptions we can share with others to enrich their lives and ours as well.

At the end of meditation today write on a card: *Oneness is the optimal view.*

Meditate in the evening as well. Review your notebook in the evening.

At the end of these exercises, if your worries about your body are in check move ahead; if not repeat them again.

HEALING HABIT DISORDERS

How many times during our lives do we find ourselves eating too much or drinking more than we would like to or smoking more than an occasional smoke? These habit disorders are a warning. We are attempting to assuage a frustration that we are not facing in our day-to-day lives. In dealing with these disorders it is important to meditate when we feel a craving for what we are abusing. If we are eating too much we meditate when we are hungry. If we are drinking too much we meditate when we want a drink. If we are smoking too much we meditate when we want a smoke. Then we focus our attention on the area of our body where we feel the craving and sit with the thoughts and feelings that come to mind. If we notice that no thoughts come to mind, only feelings of anxiety, then we can use the anxiety exercises above. If we feel depression we can use the depression exercises above. If our compulsive eating, drinking, or smoking covers worries about our body we can use the exercises above for that. The key is to find out what lies behind our compulsive activity. To do that we must sit with the craving until we uncover the symptom below it.

In habit disorders journaling is especially useful. If each time you eat, smoke, or drink you write just before you engage in the target behavior what you think and feel and just after you engage in the target behavior exactly what you ate, smoked, or drank you will make a major inroad into understanding the behavior. Several examples come to mind with other behaviors. At Columbia Hospital, The Behavioral Medicine Center became the center for utilization management for our outpatient mental health benefits provided by the hospital's insurance program. Just by asking treating psychiatrists to write down their goals for therapy and having them discuss them with a member of our staff we decreased utilization by 23 percent. In the process we never denied one treatment plan. All we did was discuss them and ask that they be written down. On our inpatient unit we did something similar. Each week we asked the treating psychiatrist to assess goals and the treatment plan. If the treatment lasted more than seven days we held a case conference. We denied no treatment plans but our inpatient utilization dropped from an average length of stay of fourteen days to nine days. Just the other day I was playing bridge on the computer and listening to a television program on weight loss. One of the most successful programs asked the participants to only do one thing: write down everything they eat. Just by the process of writing down everything they ate and coming to a once-a-week group where they discussed their experience, participants were able to modify their weight significantly. In each case having someone to talk over your notes with is very important. At Columbia Hospital we use our nutritionists for these meetings. I have my weekly meeting with my nutritionist, Peg Mayer, to look at my journal with me. Mainly we work on diet but since diet includes all nourishment, Peg does nothing to discourage talking about drinking and smoking as well.

Tom was sitting with the senior partner in his law firm, having lunch at a local restaurant, when the partner's son, a lawyer in another firm, passed their table. He asked his father if he was going to the family lake house that weekend. The senior partner said that he planned to be there and that he hoped his son and family would find some time to be at the lake too. His son indicated that they might do that. Tom was aware of feeling happy for the senior partner and his family. That evening Tom got drunk. The next morning he wondered why he had done that. The next evening when he was again craving a drink he sat with the feeling. He remembered the interaction between the senior partner and his son. Instead of feeling happy he was aware of feeling angry at the senior partner for not extending an invitation to him. He remembered how he and his father shared an interest in fishing and had enjoyed doing that together before his father died five years before. He felt angry at his father for leaving him and depriving him of the opportunity of being with him at this stage in his life. When he was able to face his angry feelings the craving for alcohol diminished.

Jim had been on a diet and had lost thirty pounds. He felt healthy and fit but the urge to munch returned and he gained back ten pounds. He realized that will power alone was not the answer so he arranged to meditate in the evening, when he felt most hungry. As he focused on his hunger the following images came to his mind. He saw a little snake get eaten by a bigger snake, get eaten by a bigger snake, get eaten by a bigger snake, get eaten by a dragon. He saw the witch's house in *Hansel and Gretel* and he saw Hansel too fat to be stuffed into the witch's stove. He remembered a time when he was a little boy and his parents left him at a camp ground, each thinking that he was in the car with the other. They discovered their mistake only a few minutes later when they stopped for gas but he remembered his terror at being left at a camp ground with big people who seemed like angry monsters to him. At this thought he felt his hunger craving even more strongly. He recognized that the angry monster was in himself and that his fury at his parents was causing him to devour things rather than to let himself feel the anger at his parents who had been so careless with his life. He let himself blame his parents and then forgive them and his hunger became more manageable.

Not all cravings are that accessible, but if we can get in touch with the feeling state beneath the craving we can often face those feelings and abort the craving.

To make an inventory of your cravings, use a notebook to keep track.

My cravings are a window to my mind.

First follow your breath. Become peaceful and relaxed. Then notice where in your body you feel your cravings for food, drink, or cigarettes. Let yourself focus on that area of your body and notice the thoughts and feelings that emerge. Stay with the feelings until they fade.

At the very end of meditation write for ten minutes in your notebook. Write whatever comes to mind about your craving.

After your meditation and writing, write on a card, *My cravings are a window to my mind*. You know what to do with the card.

After meditation feed the craving with something healthy. Feed your hunger with a nutritious snack or meal. Feed your thirst with cool, clear water. Feed your desire for smoking with deep breathing. Feel grateful for the opportunity to exercise a healthy choice, one you were not even aware of before you let yourself be aware of your craving.

Meditate in the evening again and review your notebook afterward. Repeat this exercise three days in a row before moving on to the others in this section.

Angry feelings begin my healing journey.

Angry feelings are good. Being able to identify your angry feelings and sit with them without acting on them is perhaps the master aptitude for physical and emotional well-being. Nothing predicts success of attitudinal healing more than your ability to recognize and face your angry feelings. In this meditation ask that any angry feelings buried in your unconscious mind be revealed to you so that you can face those feelings in your peaceful meditation without acting. Ask for the strength to sit with your angry feelings until they subside because if you do not attempt to avoid these feelings they will subside and then will no longer stimulate cravings.

At the very end of meditation write whatever comes to mind about angry feelings.

After your meditation and writing write on a card, *Angry feelings begin my healing journey.* You know what to do with the card.

Meditate in the evening again and review your notebook afterward.

Forgiveness paves the road to peace of mind.

Today, remind yourself of the power of forgiveness. Remember that forgiveness is mostly for yourself although it is bound to change your demeanor so it will help anyone you have contact with as well. Forgiveness just means being willing to give up the burden of resentment. But remember you cannot do this yourself. You need help from the guiding force within you. Also, remember that first you must blame, even if only for an instant, before you can forgive someone, so blame away. Search for any resentment toward anyone in your life past or present. See if there is some anger toward someone who has disappointed you. Let that resentment build. Then as you let yourself feel it, it will dissipate because emotions come and go. When it is gone, ask for the power to forgive those persons you blamed. That is, ask for the power to let go of the residual resentment left behind from your angry feelings. There is nothing wrong with feeling and thinking blame. It is only trying to push blame out of mind that is a problem because pushing blame out of mind is a surefire way to keep anxiety around. So open yourself to blaming thoughts and feelings. Anxiety is the signal that mobilizes the forces of the mind to push blame out of mind. Blame is good because it is the first step to peace of mind.

After meditation write on the card you will carry today, *Forgiveness paves the road to peace of mind.*

Meditate in the evening as well. Review your notebook and make any additions to those you wish to blame in the notebook.

Oneness is the optimal view.

Our cravings are an attempt to nourish ourselves independently of those around us. Frequently these forms of cravings do more to separate us from others than to bring us together. If we could see the outcomes of our actions on others we might be more careful. If a parent drinks too much and alters his state of consciousness so that he is not available to his child, that person will have to mature independently of the drinking parent's input. A parent's best thinking can be of great assistance to a child growing up. Sometimes a cigar or cigarette works as a blockade to keep others away or to reduce our attentiveness to them. Similarly, overeating reduces our attentiveness and may build a physical barrier between us and others.

To break down those barriers and to enrich our availability to others we may choose to see our connections to others, how much they mean to us, and how much we wish to be there for them rather than to be anesthetized by indulgence of our cravings. Today take this opportunity to extend yourself in kindness to someone in distress. Celebrate the community of man.

At the end of meditation today write on a card: *Oneness is the optimal view.*

Meditate in the evening as well. Write and review your notebook after each meditation.

If your cravings are under control move on; if not, repeat these exercises. Do the first exercise for several days in a row before doing the others.

OPTIONS FOR PSYCHOLOGICAL AND PHARMACOLOGICAL INTERVENTIONS

If your feelings of anxiety and depression, worries about your body, or excessive cravings have not improved significantly after four weeks of working with meditation, go back to your therapist or psychiatrist for help. Do not hesitate to use psychopharmacological help. Benzodiazapenes can be very useful for short-term treatment of anxiety. For longer-term treatment of depression and anxiety, selective serotonin re-uptake inhibitors are a new broad-spectrum treatment. I prefer to start patients on sertraline because of its very short half-life. If there are untoward side effects, which happens very infrequently, the medication is out of your body in just a few days.

Whatever help you get, be it psychotherapy or psychopharmacology, or both, use meditation as your protective maintenance program. That program is described in the next section.

Part IV:
A Protective Maintenance Program

This part of the book is dedicated to recharging the momentum of therapy in your life by helping you build a meditation program. It is called a protective maintenance program and not a preventive maintenance program because we cannot prevent symptoms from returning but we can protect against their lingering as a distraction. The practice routine I suggest can be done in minutes a day several times a week.

ESTABLISHING A PRACTICE ROUTINE

The practice routine I suggest is to set aside twenty to thirty minutes in the morning. Do this four to seven days a week. Establishing this routine may be met with inner resistance, but *just do it!* You will experience such rewards that if you sustain practice for just one week, the rest will happen from your own sense of progress. Let your practice build on your success. This practice has four parts that you can adopt to increase the level of effort in your practice. Reading a lesson a day and writing it on a card to look at several times a day is level one effort. Reading plus meditation constitutes level two effort and is the optimal level for most of us. Level three effort includes all of level two plus writing an example of using the lesson for the day each day. Level four effort includes all of level three plus journaling Disruptions, Dreams, and Dilemmas. You can adjust your level of effort in practice by choosing which components to include in your practice. Choose the level of effort that is most comfortable for you and at different times try different levels of effort just to sample the rewards possible at those levels.

Level 1: Reading and looking at your card during the day

Begin your morning session with a short reading. For starters read one of the goals of psychotherapy from the lessons that follow. At the end of the reading practice a lesson. Write the lesson for the day on a 3-by-5 card that you look at several times throughout the day. Each time you look at the lesson, be still for a minute and listen to your inner guide.

Level 2: Meditation plus level 1

After you have written the lesson on a 3-by-5 card, prop the card up in front of you and begin a period of meditation. Save this card because the second time through the lessons you may use the card again. Also, it is on this card that you may choose to write an example of using the lesson of the day.

The idea that meditation might be an optimal condition for self analysis came to me, as I mentioned, one afternoon in New York after a meeting of the Committee on Psychoanalytic Education of The American Psychoanalytic Association. Several colleagues who were at that meeting with me said that they were meditating daily. One friend, Larry Inderbitzen, said that he had been meditating as a way to correct a mild case of hypertension. His physicians were skeptical enough to measure his blood pressure by a special monitor that he wore twenty-four hours a day. Not only was his blood pressure under superb control but it was lowest when he was meditating and when he was conducting psychoanalysis.

This made sense to me. When we conduct psychoanalysis, we analysts are in a meditative state, that is, our attention is riveted to what is going on at the moment. We are following the analysand's process of thought without judging it and with as close attention to that process, in the here and now, as we can muster. Surely there are moments when our attention goes momentarily to our thoughts and theories, but as quickly as we can become aware of that, we focus back on the spoken words of the analysand at the moment. This attention to the moment in psychoanalysis is very similar to what we attempt in meditation. It is also the attention we attempt to teach the analysand. We try to teach the analysand to observe her thoughts and feelings without judging, as they emerge in that moment. I believe that when we lose our gains made in psychotherapy what we have really lost is our ability to observe our thoughts and feelings without judging them. I think this is even more important than any repression of the cognitive content of our psychotherapeutic work. So what we must regain is that ability to choose an observing capacity over action in a state of emotional urgency, or as it is often called in meditation literature, a witness capacity. (See the instructions for meditation on page 20.)

In meditation practice sit quietly and focus on your breath. When other thoughts come to mind, notice them and return to your breath. In doing this you are practicing your two most important mental functions, observing and choosing. If a strong emotion or strong physical sensation comes to mind stay with that emotion or physical sensation until it passes. Then return to your breath. Remember that the goal of meditation is not to empty your mind of thoughts and feelings. It is to change your relationship to your thoughts and feelings from being compelled to act on them to being able to observe them and being able to choose to return to your preferred focus of attention, the present moment and your breath.

Although you attempt to calm your mind during meditation to get below the surface noise of your thoughts, there is always something going on in your mind worth noticing. In between returning to your breath or while just following your thoughts, insights will happen, just as they did when you were in psychotherapy. They will happen as you attempt to follow your breath or follow your thoughts. They will occur spontaneously. Sometimes they will come frequently, sometimes not, but they will come if you give yourself a regular time to practice and follow your breath and thoughts. One important point is that insights come when we least expect them. They can be facilitated by asking for something such as: "I have no idea what to do about my philosophy class. I do not have time to adequately prepare for it today. Please help me find the time."

Frequently, during the day, the time for preparation will appear.

Often inspiration comes immediately after meditation, as in the case of my friend Dan Steininger, as I mentioned before. Sometimes they come hours after meditation, but they do come.

The experience of insights is a creative exercise that occurs when we are receptive. Sometimes a picture or the memory of a dream will lead to insight. Sometimes insights will occur from out of nowhere. If you practice, they will come.

Efforts to increase the level of involvement in doing the exercises

Although not everyone will wish to take the time to write in a journal, some of us find journaling the most rewarding way to nail down our gains and our questions. If you are helped by journaling, then these additional efforts may be worth your attention, time, and energy.

Level 3: Write an example of using the day's lesson plus level 2

At the end of the day write on your 3-by-5 card one example of having used the lesson for the day.

Try to remember the smallest incident of the day in which you practiced your lesson, because each journey begins with a single step, and single steps are the building blocks to inner peace. If you can master the little disruptions, it will be easier to deal with the major conflicts. This is the chance to use your creative energy to find a way to implement the lesson for the day. Even if you do not implement your lesson for the day, you can use your creativity at the end of the day by imagining a way that you might have used the lesson or imagining a time in the future when you may use the lesson. Write that story. Writing the story is a way of getting your creative juices flowing. It also gives you an opportunity to put your thoughts into words. Putting words to your thoughts helps you feel mastery over them. As an example:

I was working on "scripts for others are a part of my childhood story" when Renée and I were about to leave for a movie. I waited in the car as she dawdled in the house. I could feel my blood pressure rising when I remembered the lesson for today and said to myself, "I can release her from my script. So what if we're a few minutes late?" I realized that I was reenacting a scene from my childhood that went on repeatedly between my father and mother. My father would wait in the car for my mother, who took a while longer to get ready, and by the time she got to the car, he was in a snit. I realized that I had a choice. I did not have to poison the beginning of our evening out. I could drop my irritation after I let myself feel it. That's exactly what I did. When Renée arrived at the car expecting me to be in a huff, I was smiling. She said, "You aren't mad?" I said, "No, you gave me a moment to meditate." She laughed. We missed the previews but were there in plenty of time to see the whole movie. We had a pleasant evening together rather than one poisoned by my bad mood.

Level 4: Journaling in your *Disruptions*, *Dreams* and *Dilemmas* notebook plus level 3

Disruptions

Start a journal. Write down any occurrence that disrupted your peace of mind for more than an hour. Write these disruptions in a separate section of your journal labeled *Disruptions*. (The other two parts of the journal, *Dreams* and *Dilemmas*, will be explained later.) The disruptions may have nothing to do with the exercise you are studying. Keep track of them anyway. You will be able to identify the repeating themes that are the most important parts of your childhood story by looking over these stories later in your self-analytic work. When writing about a disruption involving a specific person make a list of the person's qualities or characteristics that you find most frightening. For instance: "Mary was sarcastic, bitter, and childish today when she made fun of my memo. I was afraid that she did that just because she was angry at me after our boss rejected my budget proposal." Those characteristics, "sarcastic, bitter, and childish," will be important later in your work. Also write the details of your fears. "I was afraid that making fun of my memo was designed specifically to punish me." Those details will also be important in tracing the themes in your childhood story.

After you have written approximately a dozen disruptions in your notebook, try this way of sorting for elements of your childhood story. Divide a page into four quadrants. Write "Men in Authority" in the upper-left quadrant. Write "Women in Authority" in the upper-right quadrant. The lower-left quadrant is for "Men Not in Authority," and the lower-right quadrant is for "Women Not in Authority."

Flip through your *Disruptions* section and write in each quadrant the personality characteristics accompanying each disruptive person in your stories.

Suppose, for example, that after doing this you have in your left-upper quadrant the following characteristics: inconsistent, picky, unreliable, faultfinding, blaming, drinks too much, fun at times, mood changes rapidly, gambling with other people's resources. Then ask yourself who in your childhood these characteristics sound like. Let's suppose that almost all of the characteristics at one time or another described your father, except "picky" and "gambles with other people's resources." Whom do those two characteristics bring to mind? Maybe your grandfather, an uncle, or a friend of your father's whom you did not like. Suppose "picky" describes a friend of your father's you did not like and "gambles with other people's resources" reminds you of an uncle. You now have a picture of three characters in your story whom you will find over and over again. The strength of their influence will be diminished as you heal these relationships through forgiveness.

Analyze the characteristics you have listed in each quadrant. The persons these characteristics describe may surprise you. One person in a group at our hospital found that the person most described in the upper-left quadrant was his mother. He was recreating his conflicts with his mother in his disputes with the men in his life. This realization came to him rather dramatically one day when another driver, a man, cut off his tractor-trailer at a truck stop. Our group member jumped out of his truck and walked up to the man sitting in his car. The man in the car turned toward him. Our group member said, "When he looked at me, I saw my mother's face." He went on to say that he knew he was overreacting and for the first time in years turned away from a dramatic confrontation. He told us, "I said to myself, 'I could feel peace instead of conflict.'"

On another page or set of pages in the *Disruptions* section of your journal make a heading entitled *Recurrent Fears*. Write the fears that come up over and over in your stories, such as: (1) fear that just when I achieve something I have been working for, everything will be taken away from me; (2) fear that I will not find someone with whom I can form a lasting, loving relationship; (3) fear that close friends will turn on me.

Do this same review each time you accumulate about a dozen disruptions and a richer picture of the characters in your story will emerge each time. As you read the characteristics of the persons in your stories and your recurrent fears, incidents may reemerge in your memory from childhood. Write these on a third set of pages entitled *Childhood Memories*. These three components, disruptions, fears, and childhood memories, will catalogue the story that you automatically bring forward from childhood to disrupt your adult experience. Just by having these details put down on paper, you will begin to recognize them as they emerge again and again in your daily life. Because you may be in therapy or have been in therapy, some of your childhood story is already known to you. This exercise will help you continue the process of discovery.

Dreams

In a second section of your journal, entitled *Dreams*, write down any vivid dreams from the night before. The best time to do this is immediately upon awakening. Start analyzing your dream by focusing on the most important emotion it evoked. Write down whatever comes to mind about that emotion, especially anything that happened the day of the dream that might have evoked it.

Then write down how any of the pictures in the dream link with the occurrences of the day before the dream. Finally, write down in a stream-of-consciousness way any thoughts connected with each image in the dream.

As you are doing this step-by-step process—writing the dream, the emotion evoked by the dream with its links from the day before, the dream images linked with the day of the dream—a synthesizing thought may come to you that will express the fears and wishes disguised by the dream. Do not be disturbed if the dream does not come together in a finished product. In that case let the meaning bubble up during the day or over a series of days.

This is a dream told to me recently:

> In last night's dream I was in the yard of the house where I grew up. An animal was chasing me and I was trying to run away but I could only move slowly as if I were running in molasses. I gave up trying to run and turned to face the beast. When I turned around no one was there.
>
> The emotion evoked by the dream is fear. I am afraid of something, but no one is there when I face my fear. I am afraid that in my latest project at work there is no one on the team with me. It reminds me of the fourth grade trying to work with Mrs. Grayson, my teacher. I would go to her for help, but she seemed preoccupied. She would say the same things over and over to me, but her answers did not fit my questions. I was trying to get help with long division and she did not understand what I was asking her. She seemed not to want to understand. I thought about telling my parents, but I thought they would not like my attitude toward my teacher, so I chose to say nothing. I felt all alone with my problem.
>
> The back yard in the dream reminds me of the exercise area for patients at the hospital. It's bounded by buildings on two sides and has fencing on two sides. It's either all shaded in the morning or so bright with sunlight in the afternoon that it's hard to be there. It's

either black or white. Maybe the dream is about my fears of working with Eleanor. She seems to want to participate in our project but at the same time she seems in her own world, hard to talk to, a black-and-white thinker. I have an important meeting with her this morning. Maybe I'm concerned that we will get nowhere, just cover the same ground again. Sometimes I think Eleanor is malicious, like the animal in the dream, but when I confront her, she seems to wither. My question is, "What is going on in my communication with Eleanor that is frightening me?"

In this case the question is the synthesizing thought. If a question arises from your dream you may choose to write it down in the third part of your journal, the *Dilemmas* section. In the evening write down any answers you feel you found to your question.

Dilemmas

The third section of the journal may be entitled *Dilemmas*. In the *Dilemmas* section write down your questions. At the end of each day write any answers that have bubbled up during the day. Put each question on a separate page. At the end of each day see if some answers have bubbled up to your questions and write them on the pages with the questions. One of the most effective ways to use meditation is to begin with a question that you allow to percolate for several days or more: "What should I give Janice for our anniversary?"; "How should I deal with Gil's encroaching on my territory?"; "Should I marry Elise or not?" At the end of the day write down thoughts and feelings that you think are pertinent to your question. Do that until you are satisfied that you have an answer. This kind of journaling can be a form of psychotherapy all by itself.

GOALS OF PSYCHOTHERAPY

The ultimate goal of psychotherapy is peace of mind through the growth of our nonjudging observing capacity, our "witness self." As we become convinced that we can observe rather than act reflexively, we see an increased number of options in each situation. The way we achieve peace of mind is to face our conflicts. In the process we will learn more about our childhood story and how our mind works. We know that much of what goes on in our mind is outside of our awareness. Getting in touch with the part of our minds that is often outside of awareness is what we are attempting to accomplish in psychotherapy and in meditation. Freud said "to love and to work" were the pleasures available in life. We might add to that to love and to work in peace would be optimal. The goals I have chosen to emphasize are ones that will help us achieve inner peace by helping us change our perceptions. A moment of healing is a moment in which we shift from a sense of urgency to act to an experience of inner peace. The goal of the lessons that follow is to help us achieve shifts in perception that bring us inner peace.

The way to use these lessons is to read them, write them on a card that you will look at several times each day, meditate on them, and journal about them if you choose to do so. As indicated above, some days you may wish to engage in one level of effort and other days you may wish to vary that effort. The choice is yours. The lessons are arranged under twenty-one headings.

1. Things are not the way I see them now.

Our perceptions are amazingly limited and distorted by beliefs held over from childhood. In addition to those distortions, scientists tell us that our senses only apprehend one part in a billion of all the information and energy surrounding us. Although, ultimately, we use our senses to apprehend reality, they must be checked over and over for reliability by the scientific method.

Does this mean that we are doomed to exist in complete uncertainty about everything? Not at all. For most practical purposes our perceptions are fine. When I look for a book in my library it suffices that I know a table is a table and a book is a book. But when high levels of emotion are involved, I am careful to check out my perceptions.

What makes this so important is that if we believe that things are the way we see them now, we cannot learn anything. We will remain stuck in a morass of uninformed certainty. Certainty is a limitation, especially when it comes to our perceptions. Later, when we discuss further the use of our inner guide, we will discover something we can be certain about, but it is something beyond our immediate perceptions.

Only perceptions tested by the scientific method can be trusted because our perceptions are amazingly inaccurate and limited. Our sight, hearing, and other senses are remarkably biased. Many psychology experiments have shown that we often do not know, literally, what we have seen or heard.

For example, returning from a trip I took my car to be washed at a car wash in Milwaukee, where I live. When I got home, I noticed two long scratches on my car roof, one down each side. I was sure that something in the car wash had scratched the roof, so I returned to look for the culprit. On the way I imagined angry confrontations and denials. I imagined a lawsuit, wasted time, and hurt feelings. Once at the car wash, I decided to calm down. I remembered the lesson *"Things are not the way I see them now"* and was still for a few moments. It occurred to me that before talking to the manager it might be wise to watch a few cars being washed. What I observed was that during the half dozen washes that I watched nothing but soft cloth ever touched the cars. The only hard surface was on the air blower, and that never made contact with any car I watched. It became clear to me that this car wash was not the culprit.

I calmed down and approached the manager. I explained my dilemma to him, saying that I was sure it had not happened here but I could not figure out how my roof had been scratched. He said, "Let me take a look." With a cloth he rubbed off what appeared to be the scratches, explaining, "When you drive on the highway at fast speeds (I had just come back to Milwaukee from New York) a drop of grease, usually from a truck, can hit your car and spread in a thread like this. It gets baked on by the sun so it looks just like a scratch but it's a strung-out drop of grease." I thanked him for his help and felt relieved that I had not acted like a jerk. Knowing that anger only arises from fear, I later reflected on what had made me so frightened. I remembered my feelings of helplessness as an adolescent whenever I had to have my car fixed and recognized that I was experiencing those old feelings. That old experience had colored my adult perceptions and filled me with fear that expressed itself as anger.

There are many ways we already know not to trust our senses. For example, our senses tell us the world is flat. We do not believe this, because we know through our knowledge of science that the apparent flatness is an illusion determined by our limited line of sight. Our senses tell us the sun rises in the east and sets in the west. We do not believe this because we know it is an illusion based upon our not being able to feel the earth rotate. It is our planet rotating, not the sun moving.

Our senses tell us that we are the center of all experience. We try not to believe that. This one is more complicated, because the experience of ourselves as the center of the universe is relentless. It is hard to write one full page without saying something that another person could barely understand because she is not inside my head. It is hard to live one hour in which I do not ask something of someone that he could not possibly understand because he is not inside my mind.

Typically I might ask, "Renée, have you seen my blue thing?" This has become a joke in my family. My wife replies, "Oh your blue thing, let's see, is it animal, vegetable, or mineral?" I expect, only for a moment, that Renée will know that I am looking for the blue pants to my warm-up suit. There is no way she could know this, but for a moment I expect her to. That is a sign of what philosophers call the egocentric illusion. That is, I experience myself as the center of the universe and everyone around me will know what I mean without my having to give sufficient information to make myself understood. This illusion is based on a belief that is grounded in my senses. Since I see the world only with *my* eyes, feel it only with *my* touch, smell it only with *my* nose, and hear it only with *my* ears, then *my* experience must be the right one. The more insecure I feel, the more I believe in my egocentric illusion. One mark of a frightened person is certainty about his perceptions. An old saying goes, "Never in doubt, often wrong."

Our senses tell us that we are separate from other people and other things. But if we were able to see on a subatomic level, we could observe that we are exchanging atoms of our body each time I exhale and you inhale, and similarly each time you exhale and I inhale. The table in front of me is slowly disintegrating and it too is exchanging atoms with me. From a distance our separateness also might be challenged if we were to see that we interact in a way very similar to everyone else on this planet. From a distance we might appear to be a part of a much bigger picture of interaction that looks like a carefully choreographed ballet. That is what is meant by experiencing connectedness. We are one. We cooperate and we depend on each other in ways hard for us even to imagine. Some lessons to move you toward this goal are as follows:

Do these lessons one each day. Write them on a card and prop the card up in front of you before you begin meditation. Say the lesson over the first few breaths at the beginning and at the end of meditation. Look at the card several times each day and each time you do, follow your breath for a minute or two.

Things are not the way I see them now.

As you look around the room where you are meditating your eyes may fall on a table. That table may seem the same as it was yesterday, but it is not. Elements of that table have changed, but your senses are not acute enough to notice the atoms that have passed from that table into the atmosphere. If you had a picture of the table twenty years ago and today, you might notice some differences. You can be sure that things are not the way you see them now.

> *There is a peaceful way to see the world and*
> *I am determined to find it.*

Despite all the turmoil in the world around you, if you focus your attention on the present you can find peace. If you listen intently to others you can find peace. Peace is a place inside you, not dependent on what is going on outside you. With meditation practice you can even find peace in a dentist's chair.

> *I cannot see what is best for me, so I put my*
> *future in the hands of the force.*

If we cannot see the world as it is, we cannot know what is best for us. With all decisions concerning the future, consult your inner guide and trust the force within you. Even if you seem to have made the wrong decision at first, just wait.

2. I am never emotional for the reasons I think because my childhood story distorts my adult perspective.

As children we made up theories to explain what we did not understand. Those theories, although forgotten, remain in place in our adult life. A recent Sunday cartoon in "For Better or Worse" shows a little boy seeing sparks rise from a campfire and saying to his mother, "Mom, now I know where the stars come from." He used his imagination to see a similarity between the light emitted from the sparks and the light from the stars. We all did this as children. Some of those theories linger and unconsciously limit us as adults. Much like the tiger who as a cub was raised in a cage with confined dimensions limits his walking to those dimensions when in a less restricted environment, and the elephant who allows herself to be tethered by a rope that could confine her as a baby but one she could easily break as an adult, so do we limit our adult behavior by unconscious theories made up in childhood.

Whenever we are deeply emotional as an adult we are experiencing something from childhood. In fact, a surefire sign that we are experiencing a recent edition of our childhood story is that we experience emotions that scream out for action.

We reinvent the people in our childhood drama over and over again in our adult life. The emotional characteristics we attribute to the villains and ogres in our everyday life come from the way we experienced gigantic and important people through our child's mind and child's eyes. We reinvent past troubling relationships until we learn to heal them. One way to think of this is that our stories are doors to discovering the lessons we have yet to learn.

We all have a unique set of emotional characteristics that we attribute to other people. When we transfer these emotional attributes from our childhood story onto others in our everyday life, we feel on the receiving end of aggression and tyranny. For example, we know we are reexperiencing our childhood story when we believe that someone is more guilty than we are and therefore we, as the less guilty, are owed something by the more guilty one.

In my drama with the car wash I was experiencing a part of my childhood story. Whenever I try to get someone to fix something he did to hurt my car, I am in for trouble. The first time I had car trouble as a teenager was when a teenage girl hit the rear of my car. Her father, a local official, arrived on the scene and convinced the police officer to ticket me. I had to go to court. It was a long, bitter tussle, and eventually all charges were dismissed, but I felt that I was right and justice had not been served. You can imagine how this part of my story makes me feel when dealing with car problems. I keep repeating that story in my daily life. Hopefully, this time I did better with it than the times before.

Like the recent movie *Groundhog Day* we are the hero of a story that repeats over and over until we get it right. Getting it right means living the story with kindness and compassion.

Each of us has a childhood story. No matter how attentive our parents tried to be, they still failed us many times. Even if they did their best, by the nature of the size disparity alone between us and them, there were times when we experienced them as unreliable, capricious, even downright cruel. We made up a drama to explain our experiences. We may have viewed one parent as a villain and the other as a hero. That may not be the same way we see them later in life, yet that early story still influences our life today. We project that early template on our present experiences without even knowing that we are doing it.

The way we know that we are projecting our story is that we have *urgent feelings that seem to scream out for action*. We feel angry, hurt, depressed, ashamed, and poised to retaliate. We are suspicious. We see ourselves on the receiving end of foul treatment.

By becoming familiar with our childhood story, we can be aware of times when we are reexperiencing it. The more aware we are of our story, the less frequently we let ourselves get caught up in the urgency to act on these emotional remnants of our childhood. We can use a sense of urgency to act as a reminder that it is time to be still for a moment and see which memory we are reexperiencing. We can sort out which feelings belong in the present and which come from the past. We can use a sense of urgency to act as an opportunity to experience a moment of healing.

When I was a child, I made up reasons for my experiences that were based on my littleness and my limited reasoning ability. These childhood beliefs distort my adult experience even now without my knowing it.

Not long ago, for example, I came home at lunch time. Renée, my wife, was at the kitchen table, staring intently at the newspaper. She did not look up as I entered the kitchen. I said, "Howdy." She said nothing but continued to stare at the newspaper. I could feel myself becoming irritated. I remembered a Christmas drive when I was in the fourth grade when I sold more peanut brittle than seemed humanly possible in our annual drive to raise money for the poor. I brought in my bounty to the teacher and when I put the grand sum of twelve dollars on the teacher's desk she did not even notice. I was crushed. As an adult with my wife, I could feel my irritation rise as I got closer to the table and Renée did not notice me. When I got close enough to see what was going on I could see that Renée was staring intently at *The New York Times* crossword puzzle. I felt even more irritated as I remembered how my father would stare at the crossword puzzle when I was a boy, oblivious to me or anything else in his environment. Then I got closer to Renée and I saw there was no writing on the puzzle. I knew that most days she did the puzzle in pencil. Some days when she was really feeling good she did it in pen. Today, there was nothing written on the paper at all. I fought back irritation and said, "What are you doing?" She said, "I'm doing it in my head." I laughed. "You must be really feeling good about yourself," I said. She said, "I am. This morning I found refills for the pens in our desk set in the den and then I went to the hardware store and found set screws that keep the door knobs from falling off the door to the basement and the door to the closet in the laundry room." Immediately I could feel her enthusiasm because I know how important finding refills for pens and door knob set screws really is to our day-to-day living. I said, "What a great day you're having." She looked up and gave me a hug. Later in my meditation I realized that I had fought off being swept away by my childhood story, and being able to do so let me have a moment of closeness with my wife. I realized that I am never emotional for the reasons I think! I cannot trust my immediate reactions because I am biased by my previous experiences. My first reactions are triggered more from the past than from the present. I project the forms of these past experiences onto my world and find these situations over and over again.

To be able to use this element of psychodynamic insight effectively, we need to spend some time mapping the influence of our childhood on the story that we create in our present experience. Those of you who have been in therapy are somewhat familiar with this process because that was a part of your therapy. For those of you in psychotherapy now, this process will be an important part of your therapy. Each time you experience a strong emotion in adult life that lingers as a distraction, you can be sure that contributions to this emotion come from your childhood. Recurring themes make up your story. When I make time to be still and listen to the force for guidance on how to return to peace and love, my guidance usually tells me to stay with the feelings and face them as I would turn a ship into a storm. The storm passes when it is ready.

Some lessons to move you toward this goal follow. Do these lessons one each day. Write them on a card and prop the card up in front of you before you begin meditation. Say the lesson over the first few breaths at the beginning and at the end of meditation. Look at the card several times each day and each time you do, follow your breath for a minute or two.

I am never emotional for the reasons I think.

Whenever you get upset or even elated, there are contributions from the past to this emotion. If you are still for a moment, you can often discover some of them. Sometimes it takes just a few minutes to gain access to the past events contributing to your current upset; sometimes it takes a lot longer. If the upset lasts for more than an hour it is worth journaling to see what you can learn from it.

Today when I am angry I will recognize the anger as a reaction to fear.

Recently Arlene, an administrator of my hospital program, told me of budget cuts in my pet program, The Behavioral Medicine Center. I was furious at her. Later, as I reflected on our meeting, I realized that what frightened me was the range of opportunities it opened. This financial change gave me an opportunity to make some changes to our program that I might not have attempted otherwise and that frightened me. My anger at Arlene was a cover for my fear of opportunity.

When in doubt I trust the force.

I was not sure how to use the opportunity afforded by Arlene's message so I consulted everyone I could think of. Finally I turned the problem over to the force, and a plan emerged.

3. Scripts for others are a part of my childhood story

Without knowing it, we bring our childhood stories into our adult life via scripts we have for other people. These scripts may take the form of *special relationships* wherein we insist that others behave in a special way toward us or else we hate them. Scripts for others may be simple or complex. A simple script may be betting one's happiness on someone's behavior we cannot control. "If only Johnny would be nice to his grandmother, then the family could be together." Never mind that Johnny is fully grown and has decided that he is not speaking to his grandmother. Investing too much in others' behavior is scripting.

Your childhood story can easily be imposed on others as a script. A script is a set routine you expect from another person, the way you want her to behave. It contains the belief that if the other person does not do his or her role just right, then you cannot be happy. Scripts are imposed in "special relationships." Special relationships come in two varieties: special hate relationships and special love relationships. Special hate relationships develop scapegoats. In a scapegoat relationship you persuade yourself and sometimes others that one person is responsible for all the troubles. Then you ostracize that person. Special love relationships are thinly disguised hate relationships. In a special love relationship you decide that someone in particular is the only person for you. That person is the only person who can offset your sense of badness. Then you make a deal with that person that he will act the way you want to fulfill your desires (your script for him) and you will do the same for that person (his script for you). Since neither of you can really follow each other's script, ultimately you fail each other. Bring in the goat. You blame him for the failure because that special person did not live up to his end of the bargain. Then you ostracize him.

When we were first married, I did not realize it, but I had formed a special love relationship with Renée. One of the things I expected her to do for me was to make sure that there was always ketchup in the cupboard. If she went to the store and did not replenish the ketchup, I was convinced that she had it in for me. It didn't matter that she did not eat ketchup on anything. I expected that she would always remember that I wanted it and be especially attuned to the ketchup supply in our cupboard. Over the years I have learned that marriage has more important aspects than ketchup, but it was difficult to learn. I wanted her to replace my mother's function of ketchup monitor.

A friend, Charley Tartaglia, recalls a similar disappointment in college when his sock drawer stopped manufacturing socks. He could not believe it the first time he reached into his sock drawer at Georgetown and found it bare. Why had his sock drawer failed him? Up until that time he had not recognized how much he depended on his mother. Instead of missing her, he got angry at his sock drawer. He had developed a special relationship with his sock drawer as a stand-in for his mother.

Some lessons to move you toward this goal follow. Do these lessons one each day. Write them on a card and prop the card up in front of you before you begin meditation.

Say the lesson over the first few breaths at the beginning and at the end of meditation. Look at the card several times each day and each time you do, follow your breath for a minute or two.

Today when I feel an urgency for someone to do my bidding, I will look into myself for guidance.

Have you ever wondered why you let some little thing ruin your whole day? One day when I came home from work my son's bicycle was in the driveway. I blew my top. In analysis the next day I looked into that reaction. I was repeating something I saw an uncle of mine do with my cousin when I was a boy. Because I didn't feel free to criticize my uncle back then, I had identified with him. As an adult I was using my son's minor infraction to vent frustration that had nothing to do with him. My script for my son was marked by my urgency to act, blowing my top.

Today I will give up my scripts for other people.

This is easier to say than it is to do, but I will use as my guide a feeling of urgency to get someone else to act the way I want him or her to act. When I feel an urgency to have others bend to my will I will be quiet for a moment and give up my script for that person. Later I may ask myself where this script originated.

Today I will extend myself in kindness rather than control.

When I feel an urge to get pushy today, I will recognize what is happening and extend myself in kindness.

Instead of attempting to force my will on others, I will let go of my desire to control and remember my goal: peace of mind.

4. Attachments are part of my childhood story.

When we make things, outcomes, and being right more important to us than is rational, we are bringing part of our childhood story forward into adult life without knowing it. The stories about ketchup and socks involve attachments to things. They also illustrate attachments to outcomes. I was attached to the idea that a trip to the store would yield the natural outcome of ketchup in the cupboard. Charlie was attached to the outcome that laundry would be done for him in such a way that his sock drawer would always be full. Attachments are made when we let things stand for much more than they really mean. Ketchup meant a mother's love. Socks meant not having to sweat the small stuff because his mother took care of it.

One day last winter our car wouldn't start. I felt panicked. How would I get around? How would I get to work? I was trapped in the cold and the snow, immobilized in this deep freeze. Renée reminded me that it was a short walk to work, or I could call a cab. We could get a rental car. Or I could simply get my battery recharged. Why was I treating a car like it was the most important thing in the world? I remembered a winter I had spent in Grayling, Michigan, after my sister was born. I was driven there to spend the winter while my sister was left with Grandma Kempf and Aunt Betty. My parents went to Florida to be alone after my father returned from the Pacific. I felt stranded, away from familiar people, stuck indoors because of the cold and snow, and without transportation. On warmer days I was allowed to sit in my Uncle Ted's car and I would pretend that I was driving to Florida. But I was too small to really drive. Was that ever frustrating! But here I was, a grown man, reliving those feelings with my car attachment. I was attached to the outcome of always having a drivable car when now, as an adult, I have more options than I did when I was a child.

Attachment to being right is much harder to give up. When my children were young, I knew exactly how they should conduct themselves and exactly how and which things they should strive for. Ah, what moments of pristine clarity! And oh, what an education I had coming to me! The humbling experiences of my child-rearing education would fill a separate book. One moment that stands out in my memory was a time when I took my two sons pheasant hunting. It was our first time out together and I was instructing them on the perfect way to hunt when two pheasants burst into the air out of a thicket just in front of us. Jeff shot at one and winged him. Michael shot the other before I could raise my gun. I was astonished. Michael said, "Dad we've been practicing with Louis Jagoe." Louis was our next door neighbor. Rather than listen to my systems approach to pheasant hunting, they had consulted a real pro. They detected my attachment to being right, so they had put up with my lecture until the birds jumped. I suppose it was not hard to detect. Attachment to being right comes when we are uncertain and do not want to admit it.

Some lessons to move you toward this goal follow. Do these lessons one each day. Write them on a card and prop the card up in front of you before you begin meditation. Say the lesson over the first few breaths at the beginning and at the end of meditation. Look at the card several times each day and each time you do, follow your breath for a minute or two.

Today I will give up my attachment to things.

Today become aware of something that you overvalue so that you can become less fearful about it. It may be just a little something. You may pass a shop and feel a pull to buy something that you do not really need. Recognize that pull and resist it.

Today I will give up my attachment to outcomes.

Today become aware of some outcome in which you have irrationally invested far too much emotional energy, such as some sports event or political debate. Start with the small things. Give up your attachment to that outcome.

Today I will give up my attachment to being right. I will ask, Do I want to be right or do I want peace of mind?

Scan your day to find a place where you are too invested in being right and calm yourself over the issue. Do you want to be right, or do you want peace of mind?

5. My sexual drives are a part of me.

Below a thin veneer of civilization, we are animals with the same two innate biological drives as all other animals. Sexual and aggressive drives are normal. Drives are unconscious, though we experience strong desires or cravings that are fueled by them. Our drives are our innate psychological forces that work behind the scenes all the time. They provide the energy for everything we think, feel, imagine, dream, and plan. They are mental forces based on a biological substrate that is beyond our awareness. These drives, when working together and not in conflict, are experienced as a smooth sense of energy. They are the mental "crude oil" that can be refined for more complex mental energy requirements.

From birth to senescence we have a driving sexual force. In the first year of life our mouth is the predominant organ of sexual pleasure. In the second year our anus takes over. Then our sexual organs come into prominence. Throughout life we have a drive for sexual gratification that must be satisfied. We have no choice about having drives. They are a given. Our decision is when, how, and, most important, whether to act on them. Some lessons to move you toward this goal follow. Do these lessons one each day. Write them on a card and prop the card up in front of you before you begin meditation. Say the lesson over the first few breaths at the beginning and at the end of meditation. Look at the card several times each day and each time you do, follow your breath for a minute or two.

Sexual fantasies are good; they are a part of me.

One of the areas where psychotherapy is most useful is helping us understand and accept our sexual fantasies. When I was a psychiatric resident a psychoanalyst presented the case of a young woman who could experience orgasm only when she imagined that her hands were tied over her head. She wondered why that was a requirement. As she analyzed this fantasy she discovered three components to it: (1) One day as she was changing her daughter's diapers she held her daughter's hands above her head as she was wiping her and saw the intense look of pleasure on her daughter's face. She imagined that she may have had a similar experience when she was a baby. (2) She remembered her interest in her little brother's penis and imagined that she may have wished to break it off when she was little. Having her hands tied in her fantasy was a visual representation of the thought: "Do not think of me as someone capable of hurting your penis." (3) She remembered her difficulty keeping her mind and her hands off her own genitals when she struggled with guilt over masturbation as a teenager.

Her sexual fantasy of having her hands tied over her head allowed her pleasure just as a baby is permitted pleasure in being washed by her mother. In the tied position she was protected from the dangers of imagining using her hands to hurt her husband's penis. In the fantasy she could defend against any accusation that she was using her hands for masturbatory pleasure.

A man who was on medication that interfered with his maintaining an erection became interested in lesbian sex scenes in his fantasy life. As he analyzed these, he saw them as a way to reassure himself that he could still have a gratifying sex life without an erection.

A man whose mother died when he was young could only have an orgasm with the fantasy of a woman as his slave. If he was sexually interested in a woman only as a slave, he need not fear being emotionally attached to the woman and exposing himself to the fear of losing someone he loved. He imagined a slave as someone who could easily be discarded, the way he had felt discarded when his mother died.

All sexual fantasies have their roots in childhood. Sexual fantasies are a way of finding pleasure through the labyrinth of desires and prohibitions experienced during the formative years.

Today be alert to your sexual fantasies. Be comfortable observing them without acting on them. In your meditation ask yourself, "Where does this fantasy come from?" See what comes to mind.

Sexuality may be refined to love and creativity.

If we can accept our sexuality and our sexual fantasies, we can refine our sexual energy for expression in more civilized ways. What starts out as a sexual attraction can grow to either include or be exclusively a kind, caring relationship. What begins as a strong sexual desire can develop into a love of music, literature, theater, writing, singing, laughing, drawing, painting, teaching, and many other forms of expression. Often such an interest will grow out of an affection for someone who helped us develop our interests.

Today be aware of your sexual fantasies and then let them move from sexual expression to expression in kindness or creativity. A goal for our lives is to be as free as possible in our fantasies and to be as responsible as possible in our actions.

6. Aggressive drives are a part of me.

Aggression may be thought of as an independent drive that propels us toward chosen goals. Anger is only one manifestation of aggression. It is experienced from a position of frustration or a one-down position. Anger may be experienced as arising from the frustration of our sexual desires. When anger is stimulated, we are driven to either fight or flight. Anger is our mind's automatic response to fears that we will not be able to gratify our sexual or loving desires. From a position of advantage, aggression may stimulate an emotion of contempt or disdain. From a position of equality, aggression may stimulate an emotion of determination, a feeling of persistence, an acuity for seeing clearly and noticing distinctions. These derivatives of aggression are necessary for intelligence. So aggression is an important drive in its own right and operates best in conjunction with libido. Aggression is necessary for intelligence and stick-to-itiveness.

Anger may be the least helpful of the manifestations of aggression but it is familiar to all of us and when we experience it, we must learn to accept it and to deal with it effectively. We can only play the emotional cards we are dealt. If we experience anger we must learn to play that card like any other.

Angry fantasies are good; they are a part of me.

Angry fantasies are a wonderful way to work out our aggression without imposing it on other people. A man who hated to hear people talk on and on had the fantasy of tearing a babbler's larynx out with his bare hands. Later in life his fantasy allowed him to process his childhood frustration of being left each summer with a grandmother who talked nonstop from morning to night, while not imposing that aggression on those around him. The fantasy led to no action. It was a way of processing his aggression without hurting anyone. It was also a manifestation of his fear that he might be put back in that difficult situation with his grandmother.

Angry fantasies are useful discharges for emotion. If we can become comfortable with processing the anger internally we will not feel pressured to impose it on others.

Today be aware of your angry fantasies. Permit them to play themselves out in your imagination without feeling any pressure to act on them.

Aggression may be refined to expansiveness, enthusiasm, persistence, and critical observational powers.

What began as a wish to hurt people who frustrated him grew into a fierce determination to excel in his profession for a man who at first was terrified of his angry fantasies. Later, as he became more comfortable with those fantasies, he became persistent in the use of his creativity and was able to capitalize on an early talent in visual arts. He enthusiastically expanded his business to become one of the most sought-after special effects companies in the country. Those special effects often included considerable violence, but the violence was in visual fantasy, not in action.

Today let yourself feel your angry feelings, imagine your angry fantasies, and then imagine them emerging in enthusiasm, creativity, and a keen ability to observe the world around you more closely. Wish to be as free as possible in your fantasies and as compassionate as possible in your actions.

7. Emotions are triggered by either love or fear.

What triggers all emotions is either our innate kindness or our fear that we cannot get our desires gratified. Unlike drives that operate unconsciously, these emotions are conscious. Drives work behind the scenes of consciousness. In consciousness we experience two emotional forces: love and fear. Love is the experience of emotional joining. Our sexual drive is the one pushing for a physical joining. When that drive is refined, love is an experience of emotional joining, a feeling of togetherness, seeing things the way we think the other person may see them. It is our first and most natural state. Anger, guilt, shame, and embarrassment are driven by fear. When someone acts angrily toward us, he is frightened and calling out for love.

Either we feel love or fear. When we act irritably, we are frightened and calling out for kindness and compassion. When we extend compassion to an angry person, we are choosing joining over separation. We are making a decision not to believe what our senses tell us, that we are separate, and instead, to believe what we know is true, that we are one. If we are one, when we extend ourselves in compassion, we help ourselves.

Another angle on this is to divide experience between two selves: a frightened-self and a loving-self. Our frightened-self started in childhood when we feared that we would not get our loving wishes gratified, so we decided to act tough instead.

Our frightened-self believes in a world of scarcity. "There is only so much stuff and I must get my share and more." It tells us that we have to look out for ourselves and get all that we can. It shouts out, "Gimme, gimme." It holds on to temporal things such as the body, alcohol, drugs, failure, guilt, depression, shame, material possessions, and money.

When we operate from our frightened-self, we make fun of attempts to explore an inner world. We believe that love is a futile whimpering of frailty. We say, "No pain, no gain." We want to drive a hard bargain and walk over other people to get ahead. We believe that anger and fear are not only inevitable, but that those emotions are justified and reasonable. In our fearfulness we attack first and ask questions later, if at all.

Our frightened-self began in childhood when we sought to prove that we could act big even though we were small. It began when we were frustrated over not getting all the love we wanted and decided that our problems must be based on our badness. Unable to tolerate the idea of our badness we put the badness outside ourself onto others. It was others' badness that caused us trouble. In other words it began with a sense of guilt that we projected onto others.

Over the years our frightened-self had a lot to say about relationships. It said that "me first" was the way to go. We should insist on "me first" even though it leads to feelings of alienation from others. When we are operating from our frightened-self, we want instantaneous gratification, with sexual gratification and physical pleasure at the top of the list. We brook no criticism. We insist on being obeyed no matter what, and despite unlimited selfishness, we expect to be admired, even adored.

Our frightened-self's standard is a double standard. While it is all right for us to act small-minded, mean, manipulative, envious, and jealous, it is not all right for others to even *think* of those feelings. If others do think of them and show them, even for an instant, it is a sign that they are not the slaves we want them to be.

When we operate from our frightened-self, we are vigilant in watching for enemies or those who even accidentally might operate at cross-purposes. "When in doubt, pout!" is our rallying cry. No slight is too small not to make a federal case of it. After all, we believe that hate is a more important emotion than love, because without hate, vengeance means nothing.

Our frightened-self believes in special relationships. *A Course in Miracles*® defines special relationships as those onto which we project guilt (Text 294–297). There are two types of special relationships: special hate relationships and special love relationships. Special hate relationships develop scapegoats. In a scapegoat relationship we persuade ourselves and sometimes others that one person is responsible for all our troubles. Then we ostracize that person. Special love relationships are thinly disguised hate relationships. In a special love relationship we decide that you are the only person for us. You are the only person who can offset our sense of badness. Then we make a deal with you that you will act the way we want you to act to fulfill our desires (our script for you) and we will do the same for you (your script for us). Scripts are the particular ways we want others to behave. Since neither of us can really follow each other's script, we ultimately fail each other. Bring in the goat. We blame you for the failure because you did not live up to your end of the bargain. Then we ostracize you.

When we operate from this defensive posture, we are afraid. We cannot help being frightened; it is a part of life. In this respect our frightened-self is not bad; it is just operating on limited information. It was formed, after all, when we were little ones living in the land of giants. When we did not get our needs met, or when we were brushed aside, those giants seemed pretty mean and dangerous. They became even more dangerous when we projected our anger onto them and experienced ourselves on the receiving end of our own projected rage.

Now when we experience others as dangerous, we can recognize this as a moment of reliving a childhood experience in the land of the giants. We can reduce the time we spend in fear by recognizing some of our options as adults. One option is adopting a belief system different from the one our frightened-self is selling. Remember, the frightened-self grows out of the fear that we cannot have our loving wishes gratified. There were times when that was true in the land of the giants. What if we did not believe that to be so true anymore? Then an alternative belief system would be available to us. That alternative is the belief system of our loving-self, in other words, the force.

Our loving-self is fueled by our inner guide, the force. The force is love and love is our essence. If the frightened-self develops out of fear that we cannot have our loving feelings gratified, then when we realize we are much less easy to thwart as an adult, we can be more hopeful about reaping the benefits of loving feelings. In the belief system of our loving-self the purpose of relationships is to join with the essence of others through the extension of caring and compassion. When we are compassionate, we focus on similarities rather than on differences. We see relationships as opportunities for giving, learning, and growth. When we operate from the force, the goal of life is peace of mind. We attain peace of mind by seeing ourselves more clearly through introspection. When we operate from the force, things that we hate in ourselves when we operate from our frightened-self are merely errors to be corrected, not transgressions to be remembered and paid for indefinitely with guilt and shame.

The act of healing is an act of compassion. Whether we show compassion for ourselves when we are frightened and irritable or for our friend who is frightened and acting like a jerk, the act of healing requires forgiveness and joining. No matter how irritable, we are connected to the force where we can find forgiveness and calming. No matter how mean they may seem when they are frightened, others are connected to us through their essence. In changing our attitudes in relationships, healing means forgiving. We ask ourselves to be a love-finder rather than a fault-finder. This is not a stance of capitulation; it is a stance of maximizing options without getting stuck in a reactive mode.

In the exercises here we do *not* ask ourselves to ignore any feelings. With a compassionate center, allowing ourselves to feel anger, hate, depression, shame, and blame may be the initial step in healing because they help us identify *where* healing is needed. There is no surer way to perpetuate misery than to attempt to avoid emotions. Emotions are not the problem. It is the attempt to avoid feelings that causes us misery. No feelings are pathological. It is our quest for actions or possessions to offset our feelings that are our downfall. If we try to find clothes that make us feel less little, then we will ultimately fail. If we attempt to keep busy so that we will not feel bored, we find that we have to slow down eventually. And when we do, we will still have the feelings that we attempted to avoid. If we try to drown our feelings in alcohol, tranquilizers, antidepressants, or anything else, we will ultimately find that the feelings are still there. Medications can be used to moderate feelings while we are learning to face them, but medications are only a beginning, not an answer.

A rule to follow is, "*No strong feeling originates in adulthood.*" All strong feelings are good because they may be used as beacons that lead us to heal ourselves in the present as well as in childhood. Beacons are to be celebrated, not repressed or ignored. Strong feelings of hate, hurt, shame, and guilt may be embraced as useful aspects of ourselves that light the way to introspective work.

With introspection the same aggressive energy that fuels anger may be loosed from past bonds to fuel useful mastery in our life today. If we can see where our anger is stuck and loosen it through forgiveness, we can achieve a moment of healing. In our meditations we can trace the origins of those feelings and let them lead us to forgive our parents, siblings, and others who disrupted our peacefulness in the past. This aggressive energy, once stuck in the past, may be freed to let us see more clearly.

However, our loving-self is slow to react. Our frightened-self speaks first. When we react, we react from our frightened-self. When we respond, we respond from our loving-self, the force. The only way to get in touch with the force is to quiet our senses and be receptive to our experience of calm, quiet inspiration. With some practice we can shorten the time it takes to receive guidance, but it still takes time. Counting to ten as a way to deal with a perceived injustice is an attempt to buy some time to access inner wisdom. Another way is to be still for a few moments, follow our breath until our frightened-self quiets down, and ask for compassionate guidance. In the quiet we can begin to experience our inner wisdom, the force.

There is a road of love and a road of fear. Which one we follow is our choice. The road of love is the road less traveled. In an instant we make the choice. In this instant. This special instant is all the time there is. In this moment we have everything we want. The past is gone, and the future is not yet here. Since there is no time but now, we have everything we need. We can enter this special instant any time we wish just by focusing on our breath. This special instant is a gift. That is why it is called the present.

Some lessons to move you toward this goal follow. Do these lessons one each day. Write them on a card and prop the card up in front of you before you begin meditation. Say the lesson over the first few breaths at the beginning and at the end of meditation. Look at the card several times each day and each time you do, follow your breath for a minute or two.

Today I will recognize that anyone who speaks in anger to me is afraid and calling out for love. I will extend myself in compassion.

This is a great lesson. The better we get at this the better we achieve peace of mind. If we only learned one interpersonal skill this would be a good one to learn. I am told that Art Linkletter had a way to get into a compassionate frame of mind when someone acted angry with him. He imagined that the person had a brain tumor. Then he found it easy to be kind and compassionate to that person. It is not so far-fetched. Sometimes anger seems like a tumor. It must be an awful burden to live with so much fear. I prefer to think of the person as having a brain abscess that may be drained by my kind, compassionate behavior.

My stressors are angry feelings that I try to keep out of mind.

Today when I feel stressed, I will look for my angry feelings and let myself sit with them without judging.

Think of your anger as a brain abscess that you will drain by letting the anger come out in your imagination. Drain the anger by staying with it until it wanes.

Hurt is hate directed at myself.

Hurt and hate are normal emotions, not feelings that we need to judge harshly. Rather, they may be opportunities, beacons that direct us to areas where healing might take place. Here is one way to process hurt: (1) Recognize that hurt is disguised anger at someone else. (2) Turn the direction of the feeling around by feeling anger at the person who hurt you. (3) Stay with the feeling of anger until, like a storm, it passes. (4) Acknowledge a willingness to forgive. (5) Ask the force to help.

Perceptions are either for separation or for joining.

When we find ourselves frustrated with another, we usually focus on our differences with that person. Then we may ask ourselves, "Are these perceptions for separation or for joining?" When we recognize a choice, we will not feel so much at the mercy of our perceptions.

8. Love is the answer.

We can learn ways to return to our innate kindness and compassion no matter what is going on outside us. When we do this, we live in peace. Finding how to return to love is what healing is all about. The Greeks have two words for love, *eros* and *agape*. Eros is the love energy that strives for self-satisfaction. Agape is the love that strives for friendship, compassion, and kindness toward others to facilitate their satisfaction. In this book when we use the word love we mean agape. When we strive for our goal, peace of mind, we are continuously attempting to return to love for love is the answer to living a full, peaceful, and rewarding life.

A paradox of sorts confronts us. If we want the most for ourselves we seek to facilitate others. Milton and Rose Friedman, in their book *Free to Choose*, explain this apparent paradox in economic terms. With quotes from Adam Smith they say that more good is done by people seeking to better themselves than is done by people who aim to help others, because by seeking to better ourselves we *must* help others. Only a win-win policy will truly be rewarded. In economic terms, only a market that rewards all participants will survive. If I set out to try to do good for others without regard for myself, I may be surprised to find an even greater degree of self-interest kept out of my awareness. Keeping my interest in mind must include rewards for others.

It helps to remember that we have two sets of feelings that determine our experience at any moment. One is love and the other fear. When love is in charge we see similarities with others and feel a kinship toward them. When we are frightened we feel differences. We feel angry, hurt, or a desire to distance ourselves from others.

John made a lamp for his den. He fashioned a long base that looked like a music note. He sanded the wood and painted it a bright blue, the color that van Gogh used for the sky in many of his paintings. He ran the wire through the base and installed the lamp in the den to surprise his wife. When Jenny came home she looked at the lamp and did not comment. John felt hurt. He angrily accused Jenny of undercutting his initiative. Jenny said that while the lamp was a true work of art, she had hoped for a more traditional look for the den. John flew into a rage and said that his contributions were never appreciated. He took the lamp out to the garage and vowed never to use his creative talents in his house again. He went to bed in a snit and had this dream. He was a little boy who had just accomplished something really great and no one would look at him. When he awakened the next morning he thought about his dream. He remembered a time when he was 2 or 3 and was in the process of toilet training. He had everything almost figured out but not exactly. One day he had a bowel movement in his bathwater. He expected to be praised for his effort but he had delivered the right package to the wrong porcelain receptacle and his mother was not entirely pleased. He could not understand why what he had been praised for so highly in the past was ignored and not praised now. His mother seemed to be at a loss to help him understand this distinction and he felt hurt and angry at being deprived of his just praise and adulation. Now he understood his reaction to Jenny. When he told her the dream they both had a good laugh and love replaced his hurt angry feelings. He could understand his mother's dilemma and love her for her attempts to help him. Love is definitely the answer.

Some lessons to move you toward this goal follow. Do these lessons one each day. Write them on a card and prop the card up in front of you before you begin meditation. Say the lesson over the first few breaths at the beginning and at the end of meditation. Look at the card several times each day and each time you do, follow your breath for a minute or two.

No matter what the question, love is the answer.

It matters very little what situation we face in life; if we face the event with kindness and compassion, it will be better than any other approach.

No matter what I am feeling now, with the help of the force, I can return to kindness and compassion.

We can learn to face all emotions. If we face our feelings rather than try to avoid them it shortens the time we feel the absence of love.

9. Listening is love in action.

There are few better ways to show our kindness and compassion than listening intently to another. Remember back to the encounters you have had in your life that made a deep impression on you. Chances are that some of those include moments that you were listened to and really understood.

Carl Rogers, the father of client-centered psychotherapy, interviewed a client named Gloria on film for a psychotherapy series made in the 1960s. Gloria was so moved by how well she had been heard by Rogers that she continued to correspond with him until the day she died some twenty-five years later. This attachment was on the basis of being really heard, once, for thirty minutes.

When I was in my internship at Henry Ford Hospital in Detroit, I took my VW Beetle into the dealership to have it serviced. As I paced in the waiting room I noticed a grandmotherly woman sitting and knitting. She smiled at me and I smiled back. She said, "It certainly has turned cold hasn't it." I told her that it seemed frigid to me because as a South Carolinian I was not used to the winters. She asked what in the world would bring a South Carolinian to Detroit. Ninety minutes later my car was ready. I could barely tear myself away from this pleasant person. I had told her my life story and I had learned a lot about her, her children, her grandchildren, her husband, and her dog, Rupert. I do not know who this woman was but I have never forgotten her. She was a terrific listener.

Listening intently is to get more detail, to let every opportunity for interaction be a chance for a connection. Four steps to good listening are as follows: accepting, clarifying, acknowledging, and joining. Accepting means not judging. Clarifying means asking questions if some detail is not clear. Acknowledging means restating what you have heard to make sure you have really heard the other person's point. Joining means remembering similar experiences that you have had. You may share them but you do not have to tell your similar experiences. Often just remembering them is enough. Even a chance meeting on an elevator can be an opportunity for connection if we are open and listen carefully.

When my son Michael was about 5 years old he came into the house after playing outside with his cousins to announce that his cousin Beckie had no idea where babies came from. I was about to launch into a lecture on procreation when Renée said, "Oh, really." Michael said, "Yes, she thinks that you find babies in the cornfield." Renée said, "Well you know better than that." Michael said, "Yes, they come from mommies' tummies." Renée said, "Exactly." Michael looked pleased with himself and went about his business. I could see how much better Renée handled that situation than I might have. Michael's inquiry sent me into a panic and I was about to cover my anxiety with a lecture on human sexuality, probably laced with as many Latin terms as I could muster to conceal my own anxiety. Renée listened carefully to Michael. She did not burden him with more information than he wanted but instead told him he was on the right track. She made herself available for further discussion while hearing what Michael wanted to know. That is true love.

Some lessons to move you toward this goal follow. Do these lessons one each day. Write them on a card and prop the card up in front of you before you begin meditation. Say the lesson over the first few breaths at the beginning and at the end of meditation. Look at the card several times each day and each time you do, follow your breath for a minute or two.

When I listen I hear the voice of love.

If we listen really carefully to another, we will discover the goodness in that person. Even if he starts off defensively, if we listen, the goodness will emerge. I have found this to be true no matter whom I listen to. Even the most hardened criminal has a spark of humanity in him under his fear and suspiciousness. Try it. Strike up a conversation with someone on the elevator about the weather and you will find goodness in that momentary encounter.

When I listen, I extend the voice of love.

When you listen with kindness and compassion in your heart, it comes out in what you say. When you extend those feelings they spread like wildfire. Kindness spreads just as quickly and surely as tension and anger.

It is your choice. Do you wish to be a love-finder or a fault-finder?

10. Oneness is an essential point of view.

If we are committed to the view that we are all ineluctably connected to each other, then we would not think of harming another because we know it would harm us as well. There is a memorable French movie, *Going Places*, that illustrates this theme. In an act of vengeance two friends saw the axle of an enemy's car. Later in the film, without knowing it, they steal that very same car. While they are whistling and laughing, as they drive along the beautiful countryside, the camera cuts to the weakened axle. That sequence says to me, "Whatever harm you try to inflict on another, you inflict on yourself." To experience the fullness of life we must feel at one with it. Experiences of separation and alienation confound us. They make us miserable and depressed. Oneness means that I am similar to every other living thing, and probably not that different at a chemical level from the things I call inanimate. When I accept oneness, I emphasize similarities rather than differences designed to make me feel superior or set apart. When I let myself feel at one with another, fear disappears. With each breath I take I am exchanging atoms with all other things. I am connected to them.

An excellent example of cooperation and dependency among people can be found in almost any object around you right now. I see a Post-it note on my computer that reminds me to call my friend Gholi Darien about golf tomorrow. Think about that Post-it note. Think about how it was made. Imagine what may have led up to its composition. There are three ingredients in a Post-it: the paper, the yellow dye, and the glue. Here is what I imagine. On a clear autumn morning three loggers cut down some scrub pines in Hemingway, South Carolina. They were using chain saws that were made for them by a group of people at Briggs and Stratton in Milwaukee. The people who built the chain saws had no idea that they were working to make this yellow sticky note on my computer, but they were. The scrub pine was sent to a paper mill in Georgetown, South Carolina where it was shredded into pulp. Into one batch of pulp was poured a bright yellow dye that was originally intended to be used in antifreeze to make it easier to see leaks in a radiator, but the dye had such a brilliant yellow color that a young chemist tried it out on paper and found that it made a note paper that you could not miss. He had no idea he was helping me remember my golf game. The pulp was then rolled into paper by workmen who only knew that it was bound for Minneapolis and nothing else. In Wyandotte, Michigan three chemical workers were marking a batch of glue that was also bound for Minneapolis. They knew the story of the glue. It was originally supposed to be used on self-sealing envelopes but it turned out not to be sticky enough for that. Yet someone in Minnesota was buying it by the barrels. It must be good for something. Little did they know that they were working to help me remember my golf game. In Minneapolis at the 3M company, these ingredients were put together to form Post-it notes. All these people cooperating together to bring me the Post-it notes I depend upon without even knowing how connected they are!

A special way to feel this experience of connection is the use of bright light meditation. Here is how it works.

After formal meditation practice, where you attempt to limit your attention as much as possible to your breath, imagine a warm bright light in the middle of your body. Hold that image of light in the middle of your body until you can feel the warmth. Then let the warmth spread all over your body. When you feel ready, let the warm bright light spread out of you to those people and things in your surroundings and even people in your past with whom you wish to feel a connection. Imagine that warmth spreading out of your body to them. The color of the light is up to you, but two characteristics are always there: it is warm and it is bright. In the moments that you feel this warmth all kinds of ideas will come to you about how much you depend on others. You will feel that interdependency and marvel in it.

Some lessons to move you toward this goal follow. Do these lessons one each day. Write them on a card and prop the card up in front of you before you begin meditation. Say the lesson over the first few breaths at the beginning and at the end of meditation. Look at the card several times each day and each time you do, follow your breath for a minute or two.

I feel kindness toward all. You are one with me.

No matter what our differences, we can approach even a tormentor with kindness and compassion. I recently experienced another psychiatrist who voiced extreme skepticism about the appropriateness of teaching self-help in a medical psychiatric setting. She was so adamant that it was clear there was little chance of our reaching any agreement other than that we would agree to disagree. As I listened to her a funny thing happened. I heard her taking issue with every component of our program that I, too, once had qualms about. When I was able to see her as someone who was voicing the skepticism that just a few years ago I shared, I began to experience our oneness. As I was able to convey that to her all rancor disappeared and we were able to discuss our differences in a collegial manner. We remain fast friends to this day.

When I forgive you, I forgive myself.

When I forgave my colleague for giving me a hard time, I released myself from all the skepticism, defensiveness, and burdens of resentment that had been troubling me. I was able to forgive myself for feeling defensive and hurt when all that was needed was active listening.

We are all connected by the force.

Since we all have a core of kindness and compassion we are all connected by that similarity. Today when you speak to others, try to experience that connection.

11. Peace of mind is my only goal.

If we accept peace of mind as our only goal, then every other objective must pass the "peace test," that is, can I achieve this objective and maintain my peace of mind? Letting go and seeking peace is a good way to derive unexpected benefits. When I let peace of mind be my only goal, I am frequently surprised by the other good things that happen. Most of the time I use this exercise when I feel a sense of urgency about something or feel myself attached to some particular outcome. I ask myself, "What is my goal here?" "Do I want ——— or do I want peace of mind?"

For the last few years Bud Pray and Curtis Bristol, two of my closest friends, have been trying to get me to change the name of a study group that we all give twice a year at the American Psychoanalytic Association Meetings from "The Mutative Interpretation" to "The Mutative Process" because they both think that the latter name more accurately describes what happens in treatment. Change does not occur because the analyst says something in particular but because a process develops that leads to an increased ability on the part of the patient to step back and observe what goes on inside his mind. Despite their reasonable request, I was clinging to the old title. I argued that the origin of the term mutative was in connection with interpretation. They argued that we do not even encourage interpretation anymore. Finally, I asked myself, "Do I want to be a bonehead or do I want peace of mind?" The answer was obvious.

Some lessons to move you toward this goal follow. Do these lessons one each day. Write them on a card and prop the card up in front of you before you begin meditation. Say the lesson over the first few breaths at the beginning and at the end of meditation. Look at the card several times each day and each time you do follow your breath for a minute or two.

Do I want ——— or do I want peace of mind?

Given a dispute in which you may be holding on to a position that might have room for compromise, ask yourself this question.

The peace of the force is with me. I am safe.

Sometimes I am stubborn when I feel threatened. If I am afraid of losing some position of dominance, I will dig in my heels and refuse to compromise. If I feel safe, accommodation is often possible.

12. I will find no value in holding on to blame or guilt.

Blame and guilt are good because they serve the purpose of telling us where healing is necessary. They are not useful to hold on to as a grudge or as depression. When we feel guilt and blame, we learn to face these strong emotions in our meditation. When we face them, we see what memories are attached to them, and when the emotions dwindle, we let them go. Then we are still, following our breath "in" and "out" as our abdomen rises and falls with our breath. We follow our breath through several cycles. We feel at peace.

Blame is pointing the finger at someone in accusation. Blame has no value in its own right, but it can be an important first step in healing. Through many years of psychoanalysis I learned to be freer to look critically at the adults who influenced me in my formative years. I remember complaining about my father's taking me fishing when he was the one interested in fishing and I would rather have had root canal than sit in a hot boat all day drowning helpless worms. One day, years after completing psychoanalysis, I was telling a friend a story about one of our fishing trips without a hint of acrimony. I was surprised how much pleasure I remembered in fishing with my father.

It didn't seem to matter that I had not been all that wild about fishing at the time. I remember the times my father and I spent poring over the maps of the lake, plotting where we were likely to find fish. The memories of our planning sessions were a pleasure all to themselves and completely devoid of the disappointment I had complained about years before in my psychoanalysis. It was then that I saw the link between my feeling free to look critically at my father and retaining pleasant memories of our time together. Blame was the first step in healing those memories. So when I think of finding no value in blame, I mean no value other than as a first step in healing, not as an end in itself.

Guilt is blaming oneself. Holding on to guilt to punish oneself is self-defeating. Yet guilt can be useful. It has value in two ways. It can be a helpful signal that I am about to tread in dangerous territory, and it can be a beacon showing where healing is needed.

As a signal, guilt sometimes brings some leftover, less-than-completely useful remnants from childhood. This signal can be productively updated in the light of our experience as adults. The signal was created in childhood and at times may be worthless. Other times, though anachronistic, the hesitation a moment of guilt brings with it may be useful indeed.

For example, I was getting out of the shower when I reached for my electric razor. I hesitated. I felt a tug from my conscience. I remembered my mother and grandmother telling me never to touch an electric appliance when I was wet. My electric razor is technically an electric appliance but as it is battery powered it is unlikely to be of danger. That was a useful warning but anachronistic because battery-powered electric razors did not exist when it was issued as a warning. However, I might be better off to hesitate once or twice when I do not need to rather than electrocute myself. So this signal of guilt is still useful to me.

One message that is not so useful is, "Do not begin a fight, but if the other guy hits you, let him have it." That was a rule my father taught me. It was not a bad rule in the first grade with a bully terrorizing my playground. Standing up to the bully was a good idea. It is not such a good rule now because it might by extension inspire me to strike back verbally when extending myself in love would be a more useful response.

The second use of guilt is as a beacon that lights a place where healing is needed. Mitchell, a talented biochemist, often felt guilty and even depressed after he discovered another chemical reaction in the brain that had not been seen before. In psychotherapy he traced his interest in observing to a time when he masturbated at the sight of a neighbor girl undressing at her window. He thought of himself as dirty and bad for his interest in the natural beauty of his neighbor. Later he experienced guilt and even depression each time he was excited by another peek at the beauty of nature in its chemical complexity. In psychotherapy Mitchell was able to see that he used his early instinctual interest to fuel his later scientific one. In the process he forgave himself for being so judgmental. He also forgave his parents for not providing him with the information that may have decriminalized his natural interest in girls. In the psychotherapeutic process he freed himself to be more productive in his work.

Some lessons to move you toward this goal follow. Do these lessons one each day. Write them on a card and prop the card up in front of you before you begin meditation.

Say the lesson over the first few breaths at the beginning and at the end of meditation. Look at the card several times each day and each time you do, follow your breath for a minute or two.

Today when I feel blame, I will let myself feel it and when it passes, I will let go.

A good way to process blame is to let yourself feel that feeling. Let yourself expand on that feeling and fantasize confronting the person you wish to blame. Imagine yourself chewing the other person out, reading her the riot act, and then when you have finished let the feeling go. Abraham Lincoln is said to have written angry letters to people with whom he felt miffed. After writing a letter he put it in a drawer, never to be mailed. Today's lesson is the mental equivalent of writing an angry letter never to be mailed.

When I feel guilt I will make note of it and then let the feeling go.

The equivalent of blaming someone else is to imagine chewing yourself out, reading yourself the riot act, and then when you have finished, letting go of the blame and forgiving yourself.

13. Forgiveness paves the road to peace of mind.

Forgiveness means the willingness to let go of blame and guilt. Although we cannot make blame and guilt go away through willpower alone, we can learn not to hold on to them and to accept help from our inner guide, the powerful force within us, to let go of them. Forgiveness involves recognizing that we have these blaming feelings, sitting with the memories that the feelings evoke, and then acknowledging our desire to let go of blame. When we acknowledge our desire to let go of blame, we turn those feelings over to our inner guide, the force, to help us put them on the back burner where they will fade with time.

Am I supposed to forgive everybody? How can I forgive Adolph Hitler or Saddam Hussein? Actually, sometimes it may be more difficult to forgive someone for a personal slight, like forgetting to get ketchup at the store. But if I accept forgiveness as a key to peace of mind, I will learn to do it well, and I will reap the rewards of inner peace. This does not mean that I will not feel moments of urgent erotic or aggressive feelings. After all, we humans are animals. Urgent sexual feelings are a normal part of the animal procreative cycle, and aggression is normal too, when we are frightened. Emotions by their nature beg for action, but as adults we have a choice that we did not have as children. We can learn to deal with our urgent sexual feelings and fearful, aggressive feelings in our minds rather than by actions, so that the amount of time we spend in an unpeaceful state is minimized. It is often more difficult to forgive ourselves our mistakes than it is to forgive others.

What does it mean to say, "Forgiveness paves the road to peace of mind"? It means that we have the power to help begin the process of releasing ourselves from the bonds of our senses and the emotions of blame, guilt, and shame. Forgiveness is mostly for ourselves. It rids us of the burden of resentment. When we feel especially wronged, we may not be able to forgive all at once or even by our will alone. Even so, we can start the process. In these situations we are willing, but it is the force that actually accomplishes the forgiving. Over a period of time and out of our conscious awareness our reasoned intuition releases the bonds of resentment.

Forgiveness spares us from carrying a burden of resentment. It does not mean that we condone the action that we are forgiving. It does not mean that we might not oppose similar actions in the future. It means we choose to let go of angry thoughts and feelings associated with some perceived injustice after we have fully experienced them, in order to restore peace of mind. Forgiveness is the opposite of carrying a grudge. It is healing for the forgiver.

When I was about four my mother and I decided to go into the back yard on a bright sunny day so I could play in the sand box in the very back of our yard. When I looked up from the sand box I could not see my mother because the yard was filled with cattle. The neighbor's cows had wandered into our yard. All I remember was feeling terrified, surrounded by these enormous animals and cut off from my mother. Years later in analysis I was trying to figure out why one sunny beautiful day I felt so angry at my analyst. I felt angry and alienated and there seemed no reasonable explanation for my feeling so angry at my analyst's silence that day. I felt angry and betrayed as if I had been promised that my analyst would be with me and she was not. I berated her for being an unreliable source of comfort. I was furious at her for her not being with me when I needed her.

A few days later while I was still miffed with my analyst, the memory returned of feeling abandoned by my mother in the midst of the cows. When I spoke to my mother of the incident she recalled that it was a beautiful day and she had started weeding flower beds around the house. When she looked up cows were everywhere. She climbed up on the porch to give her a better view of the back yard, and I was nowhere to be seen. And then out of the corner of her eye she saw me pushing my way through the cattle to get to the porch and her. She got to me and picked me up.

This memory came to me in analysis and helped me understand several incomprehensible aspects of myself. One was that each year in springtime, on a beautiful sunny day, I had a terrible day. It seemed like the weather beckoned me outdoors, but I was suspicious and angry at mother earth as if she was about to play a trick on me, lulling me into a state of decreased vigilance so that I might end up feeling alienated and unhappy. It occurred to me that I was reexperiencing an affective memory of this springtime childhood experience.

By blaming my analyst and then my mother in my psychoanalysis I put myself in a position where it was possible to forgive them and be relieved of the burden of my resentment. Every year I seem to have the same experience in springtime but now instead of feeling like the sky is falling for several days, I am aware of the return of my childhood memory and use that day to forgive my mother for the times in childhood when I experienced her as not there for me. It cuts short my "spring fever" and gives me new freedom from resentment.

One of the morals of that story is that you cannot really forgive someone that you have not blamed. So blame comes first. Blame is important because it tells us where healing needs to happen. First I let myself feel the blame, and when that feeling has passed, I forgive.

Some lessons to move you toward this goal follow. Do these lessons one each day. Write them on a card and prop the card up in front of you before you begin meditation. Say the lesson over the first few breaths at the beginning and at the end of meditation. Look at the card several times each day and each time you do, follow your breath for a minute or two.

Forgiveness paves the road to peace of mind.

Blame is an important signal of where forgiveness is needed. Find someone to forgive today. Pick out the person who irritates you the most. First, let yourself feel the blame and then, when the feeling has passed, forgive. Let the burden of resentment slip away. You cannot forgive by will alone. What you can do is be willing to forgive, but then you turn the process over to your inner guide to accomplish the release out of your awareness slowly over time.

Forgiveness releases me as much as the one I forgive.

Forgiveness is for the forgiver more than anyone else. The person whom you forgive probably does not even know that he is being forgiven. *You* know, though, because after your inner guide has worked on the problem for a while, you feel less burdened. Today pick out someone to forgive. Blame that person first and then when the feeling passes, acknowledge your willingness to forgive and turn the rest of the process over to your inner guide.

Today I will forgive my mother.

We all have some resentments toward our parents, especially our mothers or mother substitutes, because we tended to expect more from them than anyone else in our lives. Today search out something that you still blame your mother for. Let yourself feel the blame, and then when it passes turn the forgiveness over to your inner guide.

Today I will forgive my father.

Today remember something for which you still blame your father or father substitute. Let yourself feel the resentment and then when the feeling passes, acknowledge your willingness to forgive and turn the process over to your inner guide. Are we honoring our father and our mother when we blame and forgive them? I think so. If civilization is to advance, we must learn from our parents, and if we cannot evaluate their actions we cannot learn. Blaming can be a first step in evaluating.

14. Now is the only time there is.

The past is gone and the future is not yet here. Now is the only time I have, and in this moment I have everything I need. When I focus on my breath, I am at peace. Living in the present is a surefire way to enjoy life. In meditation when we get swept along by plans, daily schedules, to-do lists, and other thoughts and urgencies, we recognize these thoughts as the superficial static on our minds and return to our breath to clear the static away.

Here is an exercise I taught myself. First I worry for a moment. When I worry, I am thinking about the future. Then I feel depressed for a moment. When I feel depressed, I am thinking about the past. Then I feel ashamed for a moment. When I feel ashamed, I am thinking about the past with the idea that others are looking down at me. So when I feel unhappy, I am projecting myself into a time that is either not yet here or has already passed. It is being in the present that I experience the force. When I experience the force I recognize that the past is gone and the future is not here. Now is the only time there is, and in this time I have everything that I need.

Try it for yourself. When you worry, you are thinking about the future. When you are depressed or ashamed, you are thinking about the past. Turn back to your breath. When you do, you are thinking about the present. The present is perfect.

I was standing in line at the bank waiting to make a deposit. I had four things on my "to do" list: go to the bank, go to the cleaner, go to the post office, and get ingredients for soup from the grocery. The bank was my first stop. Only this stop was turning into a marathon. There was just one window taking customers and the customer at that window seemed engrossed in some complicated transaction. He occasionally turned away from the clerk he was talking to and let out a deep sigh. I could tell that I might be here for some time. I was feeling my tension rise and my biological response was to put my body on red alert. I have trained myself to recognize when this happens and a warning light goes off in my head. Now I knew that I had a choice. This is the only time I have. How do I choose to use it? I can feel frustrated and angry and get myself all worked up, or I can see this time as an opportunity. I chose to see the opportunity. I asked myself, "What is this opportunity for?" I decided that since I was rushing around doing errands this must be an opportunity to use my meditation skills. I chose to meditate. As I focused on the moment all the tension left my body. I focused on my breath and I felt peace. A few minutes later I was at the teller's window. She apologized for the long wait. I said, "No problem, I used the time to relax. I needed to do that because I was rushing around in a frenzy." She looked at me and smiled, "I ought to learn to do that." "You can," I smiled, reached into my briefcase and gave her a brochure to our HealthQuest Program, our meditation, Tai Chi Chuan, and attitudinal healing programs at Columbia Hospital that physicians describe as adjuncts to traditional medical therapies.

Some lessons to move you toward this goal follow. Do these lessons one each day. Write them on a card and prop the card up in front of you before you begin meditation. Say the lesson over the first few breaths at the beginning and at the end of meditation. Look at the card several times each day and each time you do, follow your breath for a minute or two.

When I live in this moment, I feel safe.

Several times throughout the day today give yourself a minute to be in the present. If you can remember to do this one minute every hour or so, it will change your whole day. Close your eyes and follow your breath. When you are in the present you feel peace.

Now I put my strivings to rest.

During the day today you will be working hard toward some goal or another. Take a break from striving several times today just to enjoy the moment. Look and see the beauty around you. Enjoy putting your strivings to rest if only for a minute several times today. If you can remember to do this every hour or so, it will make your whole day more peaceful.

15. Healing is my choice to make.

Healing has two components. One is intrapsychic and one is interpersonal. Intrapsychically, healing is a shift in perception that permits me to feel peace of mind. When I focus my attention on the present, I feel at peace. Try it for yourself. Focus all your attention on your in-breath and then your out-breath through three breath cycles. What do you experience? Peace.

Healing is a crucial part of all psychotherapy. It allows us perspective. It helps us appreciate that no matter how bad things may have been in the past, the present is perfect. If we can live in this moment we have everything we need.

Interpersonally, healing begins as a shift in perception that allows me to feel peace of mind that I extend to another through kindness and compassion. This extension of love and compassion to someone who is having a bad day is as healing for me as it is for the other person. When we extend love and compassion from that inner, center part of ourselves to another human being, we are renewing a connection. We are reinforcing a source of affection and inspiration. We are giving our inner essence, with the knowledge that whatever we give, we also receive. We know that our compassion has been received when we can begin to feel warmth come back.

This process, the extension of love, compassion, or a moment of healing, is the opposite of projecting our stories on the world around us. If we can become good compassion extenders, we will be able to reduce the time we spend as projectors of our childhood story.

The feeling of shame, on the other hand, is a hallmark of reexperiencing our childhood stories. Shame always contains a belief in our smallness and others bigger looking down on us. Shame is an intensely felt belief that we have displayed ourselves in a way that has stimulated condemnation in others. This is a potentially debilitating emotional state. Many times in the face of shame we may wish to lash out at others rather than face our own self-condemnation. When we are respectful, we "cool our jets" and recognize that shameful actions do not exist; they are merely errors that need correction. We can correct our errors by gently forgiving ourselves and asking for guidance from the force.

Not long ago Renée and I were returning from a weekend with my sister Barbara and her husband Dale. We had been with her and wonderful friends in Grosse Ile, Michigan. We enjoyed the weekend with Tom and Beth Iverson, and Bill and Sue Ervasti. They are more fun than any group of golfers you can imagine. We do not take the game too seriously and we laugh a lot. We had played golf and enjoyed the weekend completely, but now we were looking forward to getting home to see our two poodles, Sam and Sarah. We rushed to the airport and just made the last plane back to Milwaukee. However, the plane did not move from the gate. We sat there waiting. Renée was not at all irritated by the wait, and I was not disturbed either until Bob, our jovial flight attendant, came on the intercom. He said, "Well, I have good news and bad news for you. The good news is that we will definitely be leaving for Milwaukee soon. The bad news is that it will not be as soon as we might like because our uncle, Uncle Sam, has some mail pouches that have to be loaded on this plane and we have to wait for them."

As Bob showed his sense of humor, I became angry. The rest of the passengers seemed to take the news in stride. Renée was busy reading her magazine, not paying much attention to the delay. I got more and more annoyed. Why was I feeling so irritable? Then I remembered a flight I had been on thirty-five years before. My father and I were returning to Anderson, South Carolina from Detroit. We had been to see my father's mother, and we knew that she was in the last stages of dying from cancer. I knew that we would not see her again and I was very sad. Because my father was having a hard time admitting his sadness, he was attempting to cover it up with what I considered an unwarranted and inappropriate joviality. I could not tell him the way I felt because I did not want to hurt his feelings. I just sat in the plane and fumed quietly to myself. The fuming served the purpose of not letting me feel the sadness for my grandmother and the frustration at my father who was having such a hard time with his feelings.

 I had not remembered that incident in years, but as I sat on the tarmac at Detroit Metropolitan Airport, it came back to me. I also knew that the memory had to be telling me something about my feelings now. My irritation at Bob was a clear sign that I was not letting myself feel something else. I was sad to leave my sister, Dale, Bill, Sue, Tom, and Beth. They reminded me of an extended family that I once had, but now many of them were gone. Rather than letting myself think and feel that, I was focusing on my irritation at Bob. Soon after that realization I let myself experience the sadness at leaving my sister, her husband, and our good friends, and my irritation at Bob subsided. I found a way to process my feelings, to get back into the present by remembering the past, and to experience a shift in perception that allowed me to feel peace.

Some lessons to move you toward this goal follow. Do these lessons one each day. Write them on a card and prop the card up in front of you before you begin meditation. Say the lesson over the first few breaths at the beginning and at the end of meditation. Look at the card several times each day and each time you do, follow your breath for a minute or two.

Healing is a shift of perception that brings me peace of mind.

Whenever you feel really miffed, you are experiencing a recent installment of your childhood story. Remember, no strong emotions originate in adult life. If you can let yourself get in touch with the past experience you can get back in the present where you will feel peace.

Healing is extending myself in kindness and compassion.

While most of the lessons here are things we do within ourselves there are times when we can extend ourselves to others in ways that benefit us and them. These are moments of extraordinary power.

Healing is stepping back and asking for guidance.

Sometimes when you experience a strong emotion during the day you will get a feeling of intensity. Step back from this urgent feeling and remember that feelings of urgency are always a sign of a return of your childhood story. If no inkling of what you may be experiencing returns to you, step back, turn the problem over to your inner guide, and wait. An answer will come. It may not come today or even this week, but if you maintain an interest in finding it an answer will come.

16. Learning is a key to peace of mind and teaching is a good way to learn.

To keep psychotherapy alive, we must keep on learning. A good way to learn something is to decide what you wish to learn and teach it. Book clubs and movie clubs are a great way to learn about human psychology. When each person takes a turn presenting his or her thoughts about something read or seen we act as students and teachers to each other.

The most important way we teach is by example. When we show compassion and kindness we are teaching the most important lesson of all.

When I was in college the first thing I read in the newspaper every day was "Peanuts." Learning was so important in college and being far away from home was so hard that I needed all the support I could get. One day "Peanuts" delivered in a most memorable way. Lucy, in her psychiatrist's booth, tells Charlie Brown that his problem is that he has no philosophy of life and that he'd better get one right now. Charlie Brown furrows his forehead and comes up with the following: "Life is like an ice-cream cone. You have to learn to lick it." Lucy rejected Charlie Brown's philosophy in her usual forceful way, which led to one of CB's famous back flips. But Charlie Brown was right. *Learning* is the secret to a satisfying and peaceful life. Circumstances in life always change. Yesterday's answers do not fit today's problems. All we can be sure of is change and that with the help of our inner guide we can solve *any* problem.

A Course in Miracles® suggests that the best way to learn something is to teach it. Teaching means living it, not saying it. Live it and you will learn it. That is what we are attempting to do with each lesson in this book.

Some lessons to move you toward this goal follow. Do these lessons one each day. Write them on a card and prop the card up in front of you before you begin meditation. Say the lesson over the first few breaths at the beginning and at the end of meditation. Look at the card several times each day and each time you do, follow your breath for a minute or two.

We are students and teachers to each other.

Today treat each person you meet as if he were a prophet with something to teach you. You will be amazed at what you can learn.

Today I will teach what I wish to learn.

Today look over the lessons and find one that you wish to learn better. Live that lesson today. Teach it by example and you will learn it better yourself.

Everything that happens has a lesson for me to learn.

Today something will happen that is not exactly what you desire to happen. There is a lesson to learn from that experience. Write it down on your 3-by-5 card.

17. Laughter is the best medicine.

Oscar Wilde said, "Life is too important to take seriously." If we do not learn to laugh a lot, it is hard to keep perspective. When we get really intense about something, nothing helps us more than a good laugh about it. Each of us has a movie that puts us in stitches. When we find ourselves overly intense, that is the time to see our movie. In his best selling book *Anatomy of an Illness as Perceived by the Patient*, Norman Cousins detailed his recovery from ankylosing spondylitis. This dread collagen disease brings with it intense pain, which Cousins was able to overcome in part by laughing every day. He found that laughter gave him better pain control than any medication did. Watching the highlights of "Candid Camera" and Marx Brothers movies, Cousins found that he was relatively pain free after a few minutes of hearty laughter. Not only was he pain free, but his erythrocyte sedimentation rate, a measure of the body's inflammatory response, went down and stayed down following laughter. We can use the same process for ourselves. Read something funny. Norman Cousins used E. B. and Katherine White's *Subtreasury of American Humor* and Max Eastman's *The Enjoyment of Laughter*. Find something that fits your sense of humor and have a good laugh.

Of course, we really do not have to look too far to find a good subject for laughter if we can lighten up and laugh at ourselves.

Some lessons to move you toward this goal follow. Do these lessons one each day. Write them on a card and prop the card up in front of you before you begin meditation. Say the lesson over the first few breaths at the beginning and at the end of meditation. Look at the card several times each day and each time you do, follow your breath for a minute or two.

Today I will laugh at myself.

Blessed are those who have learned to laugh at themselves, for they shall have an endless source of amusement.

*Today I will step back from intensity
and find humor.*

When you are caught up in the intensity of the moment, kick back and lighten up. Find a funny story like this one: After six years in analysis my analyst finally spoke. He said something that brought tears to my eyes: "No habla inglés."

18. Today I will extend myself in kindness.

One of the best ways to ensure that you have a good day is to extend yourself in some random act of kindness. It does not have to be a big deal. Just helping someone with directions can uplift your spirits. Someone asked Carl Menninger what he would do if he thought he was about to have a nervous breakdown. He said, "I would run as quickly as I could out into the street and try to help someone." There is one sure way to find peace of mind and that is to try to be of assistance to someone else.

When I first came to Columbia Hospital in Milwaukee I noticed something very unusual. Jo Ann Ratcheson, a vice-president at Columbia Hospital, was helping first one patient and then another find his way to the cafeteria or X-ray or the chapel. But Jo Ann was not the only one. Many Columbia employees pitched in immediately to help anyone who looked puzzled in the hallways. What a wonderful opportunity to get ourselves going during the day. Seize the chance to help someone else.

Some lessons to move you toward this goal follow. Do these lessons one each day. Write them on a card and prop the card up in front of you before you begin meditation. Say the lesson over the first few breaths at the beginning and at the end of meditation. Look at the card several times each day and each time you do, follow your breath for a minute or two.

Today I will extend myself to help a loved one.

Sometimes we overlook a simple way to help a loved one, such as taking the garbage out, fetching the newspaper, or doing something someone else routinely does for us.

Today I will extend myself to help a co-worker.

Try this: get a cup of coffee for a co-worker. Bring a treat for a friend. Do something unexpected. Extend yourself in kindness. Do not wish for thanks. Let the act of kindness be its own reward.

Today I will extend myself to help a stranger.

If you see someone lost in your building extend yourself by offering to help. Find a safe way to extend yourself to help a stranger today. A friend of mine, Father Malcolm, told me that the best way he found to help a stranger was to go down to Saint Ben's here in Milwaukee and to volunteer time feeding the homeless. Sometime after he told me this I read an article that had proven ways to help a bad mood. Feeding the homeless at a shelter was one of the ways listed as most powerfully inducing positive mood alteration.

19. Today I will speak from a compassionate heart.

If you want to make your whole day better, decide that today you will feel inner peace before you speak. You will be amazed at the impact your calmness can have on other people. You will spread peace wherever you go.

I have known some people who are extremely good at this. One of my colleagues, Steve Steury, is known for the calming influence he has on the most strident opponents in meetings. He simply calms himself, and everyone else in the meeting seems to calm down with him. He speaks slowly, in a conciliatory way. He emphasizes similarities rather than differences. It has a hypnotic influence on those around him. Find someone in your memory bank who was good at calming. Emulate that person today.

In order to be successful at this, you have to give up some things that can be pleasing. At times it's fun to make a smart remark or get the last word in. Today you will have to give up those pleasures to find peace. There are some risks in smart remarks and getting the last word in. Watch the character of Aaron in the movie *Broadcast News*. We first meet Aaron when he is giving the valedictory speech at his high school graduation. As a prodigy he is graduating several years early. He says that his classmates made his last few years a living hell, and he hopes the students will be more sensitive the next time they meet someone like him, their mental superior. In the next scene we see the results of his provocations. Three ruffians beat up Aaron while he, true to form, tries to get in the last word. The bullies tire before Aaron's tongue does. As a parting shot Aaron screams, "These wounds will heal but here is something that will never go away . . . none of you will ever make more than $19,000 a year, you will never enjoy writing a well-turned phrase . . . and you will never leave south Boston, while I will see the whole damn world!" The ruffians walk away, but as they do one turns to the other and says, "Hey, $19,000 a year . . . not bad." A title emerges under Aaron's image: "Future Network News Correspondent."

Aaron's insensitivity to others hurts him more than anyone else. One might speculate that he comes from a background where getting in the last word is highly valued. One might also speculate that Aaron is not expecting retaliation for smart remarks, a costly miscalculation because despite all his intelligence and talent, his tendency to misunderstand the interpersonal consequences of his biting comments ruins his chances to be a network anchor. He cannot learn that some sensitive people never forgive a smart remark about their receding hair lines, for example. He misses no opportunity to use his intelligence, mostly with men, in ways that do not endear him to them. He is so sure that he will be hated (he thinks for his intellect but actually for his biting remarks) that when he gets his big chance to anchor the weekend news, he develops a bad case of the "flop sweats," sweating so profusely that he looks like he might flop over at any moment. He appears pitiful to the network higher-ups. He sees the handwriting on the wall and takes a local anchor job in a smaller market, a part of the "whole damn world" his earlier prediction did not anticipate. His fear caused him a world of hurt.

We all have some Aaron in us, but today when we feel that part of us asking to be heard we will listen to it but not speak from it.

Some lessons to move you toward this goal follow. Do these lessons one each day. Write them on a card and prop the card up in front of you before you begin meditation. Say the lesson over the first few breaths at the beginning and at the end of meditation. Look at the card several times each day and each time you do, follow your breath for a minute or two.

Today when I speak, I speak in peace.

Let every word you utter today come from the source of kindness and compassion within you. Be at peace before you speak.

Today when I am tempted to react I will wait until I can respond in peace.

Start with the first words you say today and make it a practice to speak in peace. You will change those around you. Peace spreads as fast as urgency. Today spread peace with every sound you utter.

20. Search out the good and praise it.

It is so easy to find fault after we have honed our skills at observation. While it is useful to be able to see error and fault, a complementary attitude is also liberating. A truly rewarding transformation occurs when we can see good and acknowledge it. It doesn't have to be a big deal. Just a thank-you for being such a good friend means a lot.

My colleague and friend, Paul Gray, is the best person I have ever seen at this. I have been in countless seminars with him in which he managed to find something good in everyone's contributions. Once in a seminar at the American Psychoanalytic Meetings in New York, a psychoanalyst in our study group was going on at length on a topic that seemed remote, to say the least, from the subject we were addressing. I felt myself becoming more and more irritated. Paul waited calmly until the speaker finished and said, "What I like about your ideas is that they all focus on the intrapsychic realm, which is what we are addressing today." It had not even occurred to me to see that connection. The speaker, who until then had seemed to be quite anxious and who had been coping with his anxiety by speaking non-stop, seemed to calm down and fit himself comfortably into the group from that moment on. Paul had been focusing on what was good about what the speaker was saying, and he praised that while letting the other go by unaddressed.

Some lessons to move you toward this goal follow. Do these lessons one each day. Write them on a card and prop the card up in front of you before you begin meditation. Say the lesson over the first few breaths at the beginning and at the end of meditation. Look at the card several times each day and each time you do, follow your breath for a minute or two.

Today I will see similarity rather than differences.

With each person you encounter today let the experience be one in which you discover the similarities between you.

Just for today let yourself ignore the differences and just see the similarities between you and every other person you meet.

Today I will seek out the good and praise it.

Look for the good in every person you encounter today. Praise the good, if only to yourself, and in your kind, compassionate manner toward others.

21. I have an inner guide, the force, which I can access in quiet moments.

When in doubt, when afraid, when in need of help, I have a resource inside me that I can access by being still for a moment and focusing on my breath. When I seek the counsel of my own inner guide, the force, I feel peaceful. If I need an answer I can ask for guidance. When I need solace, I can ask for peace. Learning to access my inner guide, the force, is the most important lesson I can learn. The quiet, peaceful voice is the one I seek in my internal dialogue.

What is this force? Manuel de la Torre, a well known golf professional, was trying to help me hit a wedge, the short iron in golf, used near the green. I asked him, "How do you know how hard to hit it?" He gave me three golf balls and then moved away from me. He said, "Throw me the first ball." I threw it to him. He moved farther away and had me repeat the task with the second ball. Then he moved farther away and had me throw him the third ball. I managed to do as he asked. He moved back to my side and said, "How did you know how hard to throw the balls?" I said, "I didn't think about it." He said, "Exactly." He explained that I knew how hard to throw the balls from my previous experience. He encouraged me to use the same method when hitting a wedge. When I am able to clear my mind and trust my memory I can do that.

A similar method is used in instinctive shooting. I remember seeing on television some students given a BB gun and taught to shoot rings thrown in the air with the BB gun without so much as a sight on it. After some practice they became unbelievably accurate, able to shoot a hole through a ring no larger than a half dollar thrown in the air. This is a practiced skill that increases intuitive ability.

We all have such a skill that we can get in touch with at times. All problem solving begins with our reasoned intuition. The more we trust this ability and the more we learn to use it, the better we can become in learning where to begin to solve our problems. The force is the intuitive aspect of our unconscious mind filtered through our mature sense of reason—in other words, our reasoned intuition. The force is the part of us that we can get in touch with by being still and listening. It is a quiet voice and a voice of peace.

Being able to trust the force is the most important capacity you can achieve because it will help you in any moment of dilemma. As is written in Ecclesiastes 9:11–12, "The race is not to the swift, nor the battle to the strong, neither yet bread to the wise, nor yet riches to men of intelligence, nor yet favor to men of skill; but time and chance happen to them all. For no one can anticipate the time of disaster." The training that prepares us to deal with our internal sense of disaster is learning to trust our own inner counsel, the force. What do we know about the force?

Here are some things you can know about the force:

- The force is a voice of love, compassion, and joining.
- With some practice most people can learn to access the force.
- All people seem to have it.
- It is similar in many people.
- The frightened-self speaks first. To get in touch with the force, we quiet our senses that pick up the noise and static surrounding us and spend some quiet time listening.
- Some people experience the force as thoughts, some as words, some as pictures, and some as a mixture of all of these.

Just use it. In order to use the force be still and look into yourself. It does not matter if you begin as a skeptic. I certainly did. In fact, it may be better to begin that way, because to accept something on authority, without data, is not wise. Skepticism will come and go like every other thought and feeling.

Not too long ago I had the rare opportunity to teach a class on psychoanalytic theory with Dr. Charles Brenner, a pioneer in the field. One student asked Dr. Brenner if he could use this theory without believing in it. Dr. Brenner suggested that belief had nothing to do with it. He said, "If you open that window and step out of it you do not have to believe in gravity. You will fall to the ground whether you believe in gravity or not."

It is similar with the force. You do not have to believe in it, all you have to do is "DO IT."

Some lessons to move you toward this goal follow. Do these lessons one each day. Write them on a card and prop the card up in front of you before you begin meditation. Say the lesson over the first few breaths at the beginning and at the end of meditation. Look at the card several times each day and each time you do, follow your breath for a minute or two.

In the quiet I feel the force.

Every hour or so during the day be still for a moment, close your eyes, follow your breath, and experience the peace of your inner guide.

I can step back and let the force lead the way.

During the day today you will encounter many moments when you have no clue what to do next. These are moments of opportunity. The opportunity is to step back for a moment and ask for guidance from the force. Let the force lead the way.

As for the future I trust the force.

If things are not the way we see them now, how can we possibly know what would be best for us? Put the future in the hands of the force. When we have no idea what would be best for us in the future we can see this as an opportunity to trust the force.

Some experience the force as the Force, that is, God or the Holy Spirit. For those who share this perspective here is a prayer from St. Francis of Assisi:

> May it be, oh Lord, that I seek not so much to be consoled as to console, to be understood as to understand, to be loved as to love. Because it is in forgetting one-

self that one is found; it is in pardoning that one obtains pardon.

FREQUENTLY ASKED QUESTIONS

Question 1. I get something out of doing the meditation but I just do not like writing in a journal. It doesn't seem to help. Should I force myself to do it anyway?
Answer 1. The guiding principle in all these suggestions is to be kind to yourself. If writing makes the work an unusual burden then do not do it. Only do the parts of the lessons that work for you.

Question 2. Sometimes when I try to turn my depressed feelings around to be angry at someone there is no one to blame. It is just a situation. What do I do then?
Answer 2. First try to see whom you can blame for enforcing the situation. A colleague of mine, Dan, was forced to retire from the Navy because of cutbacks in the military. He knew that it was no one's fault, just a sign of the times. But he decided to blame the President in his meditation. Not that the President was solely to blame, but in meditation we do not expect to blame the right person. We are using the person we blame as a scapegoat because in truth there is never one person to blame for anything. This therapeutic scapegoating is just a step toward forgiveness, which is the healing function. How can you forgive if you do not blame someone first? So just pick out a scapegoat and blame him. One friend of mine picks out an old scapegoat from high school and concocts a story about how his current troubles are all Allen Myer's fault. When in doubt he blames Allen for everything. Specificity need not be an

issue in blaming. Allen may be the most forgiven person in my high school class.

In the final analysis the only thing to blame is our limited perceptual ability because we cannot see how things go together. I recently read in *The New York Times Book Review* a critique by Ed Regis of *The Pinball Effect*, by James Burke, the author of *Connections*, in which Burke links the introduction of spices from the Middle East to various hot pickling processes to the invention of electricity, the laser, and, ironically, smart bombs, which when used in the Persian Gulf War were called by the code name "pickle" and when armed were said to be "hot pickles." Now it would be impossible for us to see such links between things happening over long periods of time so when we attribute cause or blame to anything in our perceptual field we must acknowledge the limitations of our capacities.

Question 3. I try to remember to look at my lesson every hour, but sometimes I only look at the card two or three times a day. Does that hinder the practice?
Answer 3. No. Experience has shown that you will look at your card as many times as it is useful to you, so whatever number of times you look at your card is the precise number of times that you need to look at your card.

Question 4. I tried different times to meditate. When I meditate in the morning I usually feel refreshed the whole day long, but sometimes something interferes with my being able to meditate in the morning so I try to meditate in the evening. When I meditate in the evening I usually fall asleep. What does that mean? Do you have any suggestions?

Answer 4. If you fall asleep during meditation it means that you are tired. Be pleased that you have given yourself an opportunity to rest. If something interrupts your schedule so that you do not have time for sitting meditation in the morning, try another time. Once you have overcome your symptoms you can use a lot of variations for the protective maintenance plan. You might try *walking meditation* during work when you are walking from one place to another. That means being calm and peaceful during your walk, counting the steps, and smiling peacefully as you dwell in those moments. Let thoughts and feelings come and go without judging them. Another form of meditation you can use is *listening meditation.* In this practice you stay in the moment and listen nonjudgmentally to what is said. You ask for clarification of points you do not understand. You restate what you hear to make sure you have received the messages sent. Listening is a very relaxing form of meditation. Remember, meditation can be practiced at any moment. When you are fully in the present and engrossed in the moment you are meditating, whether you are sitting in the quiet, working in the garden, carrying wood, walking on a treadmill, rowing a *HealthRider*, skiing on a *NordicTrack*, or following the lyrics to a Beatles tune. You do not have to force anything into or out of your mind in meditation; just watch what happens without judging it.

Question 5. I just cannot keep my mind blank. It makes me so frustrated.
Answer 5. Remember, the purpose is not to keep your mind blank of thoughts and feelings. The purpose of meditation is to reestablish what we had when we were in psychoanalysis or psychotherapy: an observing ego, which

is a part of our mind that can observe our thoughts and feelings without judging them, without acting on them, and without using them immediately as planned action. So, it is good that you cannot keep a blank mind. A blank mind is not what we are looking for in this type of meditation because a blank mind would not be training your observing capacity.

Part V: Keeping It Going

LISTENING WITH YOUR SIGNIFICANT OTHER

If you are married or have a significant other you already have the makings of a study group. In some ways a marriage is an ideal study group, especially if both of you have been in therapy and therefore already have a background in psychodynamics. Sometimes, though, a spouse does not feel comfortable working on this project or has a different priority. In that case it is important to remember that peace of mind is your only goal and do not impose a script on your spouse. Another option is to get a group of friends together to give this a try. Take an introductory meditation class together and then meet once a week to meditate and work on the lessons in this book. Meditation classes are given almost everywhere these days. Any center that teaches mindfulness meditation or analytic meditation will give you the background you need to begin practice.

FORMING A STUDY GROUP

Here is the way I suggest you structure a study group. First there needs to be a designated leader in each group. The leader may have some special training for running a group or just be suited by temperament to keep on track with kindness and tact. When the group meets follow this format:

1. Begin by giving each member a chance to share an example of using a specific lesson in the book to achieve a shift in perception that brought peace of mind. If a participant does not have an incident to relate she may pass.
2. The second time around the group, the leader limits participation to discussion of lessons that participants are finding hard to implement. Listen attentively. If another has shared the difficulty but found a way to deal with it this is the time to share.
3. The third time around the group, discuss each participant's experience with meditation. Exchange useful tips.
4. Use the rest of the time in meditating together.

There is only one activity to be avoided. *Stay away from giving advice on how to live one's life.* Each person is his own expert in that. And the answer to any question about how to live life is to look into oneself and trust the force.

OTHER RESOURCES

If you are unable to start a study group, call the Network for Attitudinal Healing International at (512) 327–4568. They can tell you if there is an Attitudinal Healing study group formed in your area.

If you get stuck in symptoms of anxiety and depression, do not forget the option of returning to therapy for a few sessions to help yourself get over a hump. Most therapists welcome this and do not consider it a sign of need for a prolonged return to therapy. Do not hesitate to ask for help. There is no substitute for a therapist you trust.

FINDING YOUR OWN PATH

While this book suggests a way to choose the level of effort you need to put into your daily protective maintenance plan, you may find a path that is a variation of what is suggested here. I have a colleague who only journals each day. I have another who only meditates each day. Many in our study groups only read and look at their cards each day without either meditating or journaling. There is no way to be sure what you will find most useful but whatever it is, it is just the right thing for you, so do it. The main goal is to develop a learning lifestyle, that is, one that allows you to jump out of bed eagerly each morning looking forward to the lessons you have to learn that day. It encompasses seeing each person in your life as a teacher who has something to offer you and therefore deserves your gratitude and respect. In turn, you bring to the table peacefulness and a willingness to listen. Such a lifestyle is an endless source of pleasure and peace. May you find it!

CONTINUING STUDY

These exercises are designed to help you begin a journey of lifelong learning. Here are some suggested routes of study:

Mindfulness Meditation is a direction that easily dovetails with a study of psychodynamics. If fact, the elements of psychodynamics may be thought of as bite-sized pieces of philosophy that make Mindfulness Meditation more usable. Here are a few of my favorite books on meditation:

1. Thich Nhat Hanh. (1976). *The Miracle of Mindfulness: A Manual of Meditation*. Boston: Beacon Press.
2. Jon Kabat-Zinn. (1994). *Wherever You Go There You Are*. New York: Hyperion.
3. Jack Kornfield. (1993). *A Path With Heart*. New York: Bantam Books.

The best place to continue reading about journaling is *At a Journal Workshop* by Ira Progoff, Ph.D., Los Angeles: Jeremy P. Archer, Inc. 1975, 1992. I am indebted to Jim Boeglin for giving me this book. It has an excellent section on Spiritual Steppingstones and Inner Wisdom Dialogue that is a perfect fit with meditation study.

Psychoanalysis is alive and well despite the reports of the last four decades of its demise. If you are interested in learning more about your childhood story and how that influences you throughout your daily life you may wish to try psychoanalysis. In many major cities there are psychoanalysts who will see patients for a range of fees. People who want psychoanalysis can find it at a price they can afford after an assessment to make sure that it is the optimal treatment. The American Psychoanalytic Association has a number of institutes and training facilities around the country. In addition, there are Division 39 institutes sponsored by The American Psychological Association, institutes of The International Psychoanalytic

Association, and independent institutes sponsored by universities, such as New York University. There is no centralized phone number for these institutes but the *Yellow Pages* often includes local listings. Many institutes have a psychotherapy program for those who want to start out more slowly at first before trying psychoanalysis.

Psychoanalysis is conducted with the patient lying on a couch. Psychotherapy is conducted face to face. Psychotherapy is conducted with one or two visits per week. Psychoanalysis is conducted with more visits per week. The conduct of the therapist is similar whether the patient is in psychoanalysis or psychotherapy. The major difference is in what comes to the mind of the patient. In both psychotherapy and psychoanalysis the patient tries to say whatever comes into his mind. In psychoanalysis lying on the couch allows more to come to mind and more frequent sessions permit a more cohesive investigation.

Here is the number of the American Psychoanalytic Association to find a resource in your area: (212) 752–0450.

Other books for continued study in Attitudinal Healing are *Love Is Letting Go of Fear* by Gerald Jampolsky and *Love Is the Answer* by Gerald Jampolsky and Diane Cirincioni. *A Course in Miracles*® is available from The Foundation for Inner Peace, Inc. P.O. Box 598, Mill Valley, CA 94942. It is the ultimate in self study courses in Attitudinal Healing.

POSTSCRIPT

The ultimate hope for all of us who are attempting to help ourselves is that we will develop a learning lifestyle. In such a lifestyle we get up each morning with an eagerness to learn from the day ahead of us. We know that the lessons of life may come at any moment and that each person around us is our teacher. We hope to afford each person the respect and gratitude that he or she deserves. If we can trust life to be our teacher then we can believe this prayer that may be addressed to our inner source of inspiration and guidance.

Dear Source, I have some bad news and some good news. The bad news is that I do not know where I am or where I'm going. Off and on I'm not even sure who I am. Past experience shows me I could not have predicted ten years ago what I would be doing now or even where I would be today. And I have no idea how long this journey will take or where and when it will end. Also, when I try to do the right thing, a lot of the time I end up causing more trouble than good. The good news is that my source of inspiration and guidance is always with me and you encourage me to see my mistakes as errors to be corrected rather than wallow in guilt and shame. And when I trust you I find unplanned and unexpected sources of pleasure and peace. So summing up, all in all, things aren't half bad. Amen.

Index

Action impulse, meditation practice, 26–27
Aggression, protective maintenance program, 107–109
Agoraphobia, symptom return, 10
Anger
 body pain and worry, 66–67
 habit disorders, 73
 object of, 43–44
 at self, 24–25, 39–41
Anxiety
 meditation strategies, 47–61
  daily practice, 54–55
  forgiveness, 58–59
  generally, 47–54
  oneness, 60–61
  peace and conflict, 57–58
  projections, 59–60
  stressors are grievances, 56–57
  teaching role of anxiety, 55
  unknowingness, 55–56
 symptom return, 9–11

Appetite disturbance, symptom return, 6
Attachments, childhood and, protective maintenance program, 102–104

Blame, protective maintenance program, 128–131
Bodily sensations, meditation practice, 25–26
Body, as window to mind, body pain and worry, meditation strategies, 62–65
Body pain and worry
 angry feelings as healers, 66–67
 body as window to mind, 62–65
 forgiveness, 67–68
 generally, 61–62
 oneness, 68–69
 stressors are grievances, 65–66
Boeglin, J., xiii
Breath awareness, meditation practice, 28

INDEX

Breathing exercises, meditation practice and, 18–19
Brenner, C., 154

Castration, anxiety, 49, 51–52
Childhood, distortions from, 93–104
Compassion, protective maintenance program, 148–150
Conflict, anxiety, meditation strategies, 57–58
Cousins, N., 145
Cravings, as window to mind, habit disorders, meditation strategies, 72–73

de la Torre, M., 152
Depression
 meditation strategies, 35–47
  anger turned inward, 39–41
  daily practice, 38–39
  emotion, 45–46
  forgiveness, 41–43
  generally, 35–38
  healing process, 41
  object of anger, 43–44
  teaching role of depression, 39
  whoever suffers is not me, 44–45
 symptom return, 4–8
Dilemmas, journaling, 87–88
Disruptions, journaling, protective maintenance program, 82–85
Dreams, journaling, 85–87

Eastman, M., 145
Eating disorders, habit disorders, 12. *See also* Habit disorders

Emotions
 meditation practice, 24–25
 meditation strategies, depression, 45–46
 protective maintenance program
  childhood distortions, 93–99
  triggers, 109–117
Energy loss, symptom return, 6–7

Fear
 anxiety, 49
 meditation strategies, 45–46
 protective maintenance program, 109–117
Forgiveness
 anxiety, meditation strategies, 58–59
 body pain and worry, meditation strategies, 67–68
 depression, meditation strategies, 41–43
 habit disorders, meditation strategies, 73–74
 protective maintenance program, 131–136
Freud, S., xvii, 49

Generalized anxiety disorder, symptom return, 9
Goodness, protective maintenance program, 150–152
Grievances
 anxiety, 56–57
 body pain and worry, meditation strategies, 65–66

INDEX

Guilt, protective maintenance program, 128–131

Habit disorders
  meditation strategies, 69–75
    angry feelings as healers, 73
    cravings as window to mind, 72–73
    forgiveness, 73–74
    generally, 69–72
    oneness, 74–75
  symptom return, 12–13
Healing, as choice, protective maintenance program, 139–143
Here and now, protective maintenance program, 136–138
High blood pressure, meditation and, xviii

Impulse to action, meditation practice, 26–27
Inderbitzen, L., xviii
Inner guide, protective maintenance program, 152–156
Insight, meditation practice, 29–31
Introspection, symptom return preventive, xiii–xiv, xvi
Intruders, meditation practice, 27
Intrusive thoughts, meditation practice, 23–24

Jampolsky, G., xiv
Journaling
  protective maintenance program, 82–88

symptom return preventive, xiii–xiv

Kindness, protective maintenance program, 146–148
Kopka, T., xiii

Laughter, protective maintenance program, 145–146
Learning, as key, protective maintenance program, 143–144
Listening
  as love in action, protective maintenance program, 120–123
  with significant other, 161
Loss, anxiety, 49–51
Love
  as answer, protective maintenance program, 117–120
  emotional triggers, protective maintenance program, 109–117
  listening as, protective maintenance program, 120–123
  meditation strategies, depression, 45–46

Mantra, meditation practice and, 22
McClintock, J., xiii
Meditation
  continuing study of, 163–165
  high blood pressure and, xviii
  mindfulness, xix–xx
  symptom return preventive, xiii–xiv

Meditation practice, 17–31
  action impulse, 26–27
  anger at self, 24–25
  bodily sensations, 25–26
  breath awareness, 28
  correct time length, 28–29
  correct way, 28
  emotions, 24
  ending of, 28
  insight, 29–31
  intruders, 27
  intrusive thoughts, 23–24
  noise, 27
  physical activity during, 27–28
  recommendations for, 17–23
Meditation strategies, 33–76
  anxiety, 47–61
    daily practice, 54–55
    forgiveness, 58–59
    generally, 47–54
    oneness, 60–61
    peace and conflict, 57–58
    projections, 59–60
    stressors are grievances, 56–57
    teaching role of anxiety, 55
    unknowingness, 55–56
  body pain and worry, 61–69
    angry feelings as healers, 66–67
    body as window to mind, 62–65
    forgiveness, 67–68
    generally, 61–62
    oneness, 68–69
    stressors are grievances, 65–66
  depression, 35–47
    anger turned inward, 39–41
    daily practice, 38–39
    emotion, 45–46
    forgiveness, 41–43
    generally, 35–38
    healing process, 41
    object of anger, 43–44
    oneness, 46–47
    teaching role of depression, 39
    whoever suffers is not me, 44–45
  habit disorders, 69–75
    angry feelings as healers, 73
    cravings as window to mind, 72–73
    forgiveness, 73–74
    generally, 69–72
    oneness, 74–75
  overview of, 33–35
  psychological and pharmacological intervention options, 75–76
Menninger, C., 146
Mind
  body as window to, body pain and worry, meditation strategies, 62–65
  cravings as window to, habit disorders, meditation strategies, 72–73
Mindfulness meditation. *See* Meditation

Noise, meditation practice, 27

Obsessive compulsive disorder, symptom return, 10
Oneness
  anxiety, meditation strategies, 60–61
  body pain and worry, meditation strategies, 68–69

INDEX

depression, meditation strategies, 46–47
habit disorders, meditation strategies, 74–75
protective maintenance program, 123–126

Pain. *See* Body pain and worry
Panic attacks, symptom return, 9–10
Peace of mind
  anxiety, meditation strategies, 57–58
  protective maintenance program, 126–128
Perceptual distortion, protective maintenance program, 89–93
Pessimism, symptom return, 7–8
Pharmacological intervention, meditation strategies, 75–76
Physical activity, during meditation practice, 27–28
Prayer, protective maintenance program, 155–156
Projections, anxiety, meditation strategies, 59–60
Protective maintenance program, 77–159
  aggression, 107–109
  blame and guilt, 128–131
  childhood, 93–104
    attachments, 102–104
    emotional distortions, 93–99
    scripts from, 99–102
  compassion, 148–150
  emotional triggers, 109–117
  forgiveness, 131–136
  goodness, 150–152
  healing as choice, 139–143
  here and now, 136–138
  inner guide, 152–156
  kindness, 146–148
  laughter, 145–146
  learning as key, 143–144
  listening as love in action, 120–123
  love as answer, 117–120
  oneness, 123–126
  peace of mind, 126–128
  perceptual distortion, 89–93
  psychotherapy goals, 88
  questions about, 156–159
  routines, 77–88
  sexuality, 104–107
Psychological intervention options, meditation strategies, 75–76
Psychotherapy
  benefits of, ix, xvii–xviii
  protective maintenance program, 88. *See also* Protective maintenance program
  symptom return and, xiv–xvi. *See also* Symptom return

Ratcheson, J. A., 146
Relaxation exercise, meditation practice and, 17
Repression, symptom return and, xvi–xvii
Resources, 162–163
Return of symptoms. *See* Symptom return
Rogers, C., 120
Routines, protective maintenance program, 77–88

Sadness, symptom return, 4–5
Sarno, J., 12, 62n3

Scripts, from childhood, protective maintenance program, 99–102
Self-esteem, symptom return, 7–8
Sexuality, protective maintenance program, 104–107
Significant other, listening with, 161
Sims, M. J., 17
Sleep disturbance, symptom return, 5
Smoking, habit disorders, 12. *See also* Habit disorders
Somatoform and somatization disorders, 11–12. *See also* Body pain and worry
Steininger, D., 22
Stressors
  anxiety, 56–57
  body pain and worry, meditation strategies, 65–66
Study groups, formation of, 162
Suicide, management of, 51–52
Symptom return
  anxiety, 9–11
  case examples, xiv–xvi
  depression, 4–8
  appetite disturbance, 6
  energy loss, 6–7
  pessimism and low self-esteem, 7–8
  sadness, 4–5
  sleep disturbance, 5
  habit disorders, 12–13
  meditation strategies for, 33–76. *See also* Meditation strategies
  overview of, 1–4
  repression and, xvi–xvii
  somatoform and somatization disorders, 11–12
  suggestions for action, 13–14
Symptom return preventive, xiii–xiv

Teaching, learning by, protective maintenance program, 143–144

Unknowingness, anxiety, meditation strategies, 55–56

White, E. B., 145
White, K., 145
Worry. *See* Body pain and worry